INSTANT
Haircare

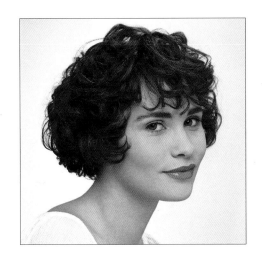

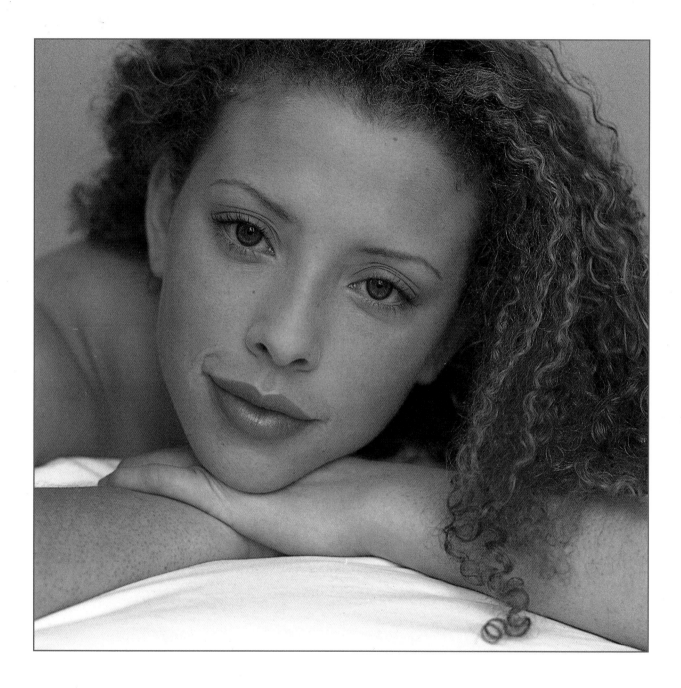

INSTANT

Haircare

The complete guide to haircare and styling

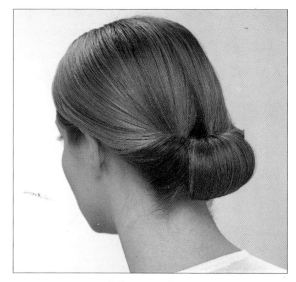

Jacki Wadeson

LORENZ BOOKS

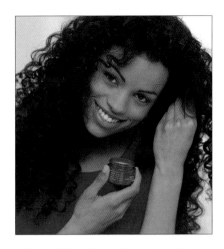

First published in 1998 by Lorenz Books

© Anness Publishing Limited 1998

Lorenz Books is an imprint of Anness Publishing Limited,
Hermes House, 88–89 Blackfriars Road, London SE1 8HA

ISBN 1 85967 689 8

A CIP catalogue record for this book is available from the British Library

Publisher: Joanna Lorenz
Project Editor: Sarah Ainley
Designer: Ian Sandom
Photography: Alistair Hughes
Hair: Kathleen Bray

Printed in Singapore by Star Standard Industries Pte. Ltd.

1 3 5 7 9 10 8 6 4 2

Contents

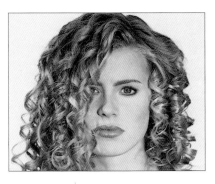
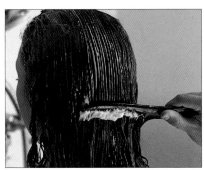
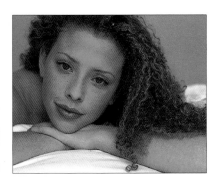

Healthy Hair

Beautiful, shining hair is a valuable asset.
It can also be a versatile fashion accessory,
to be coloured, curled, dressed up or smoothed
down – all in a matter of minutes. However, too
much attention combined with the effects of a poor
diet, pollution, air-conditioning and central heating
can mean that your hair becomes the bane of your
life rather than your crowning glory. A daily haircare
routine and prompt treatment when problems do
arise are of vital importance in maintaining
the natural beauty of healthy hair.

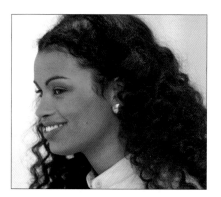

Above: Individual hair types need
individual treatments: adopt a personal
routine to keep your hair at its best.

Right: Healthy hair reflects well-being
and has a natural beauty of its own.

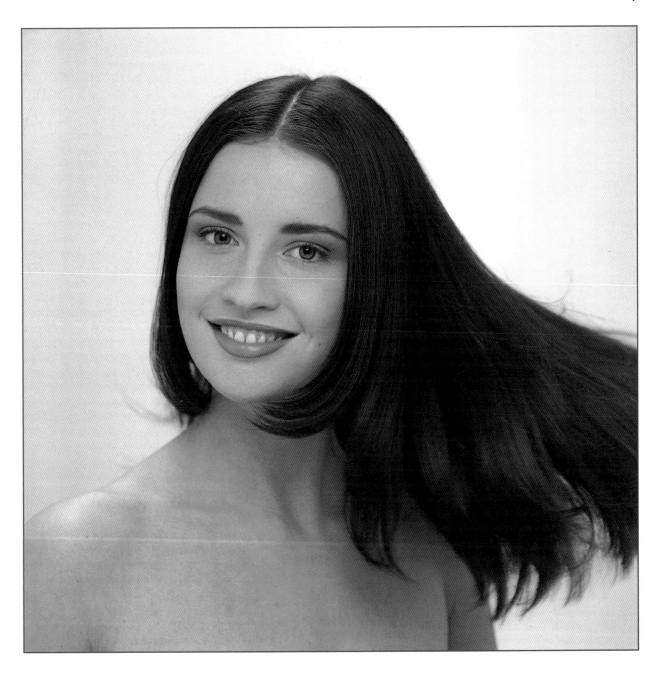

What is Hair?

Human hair is made up of a protein called keratin, as well as some moisture and the trace metals and minerals found in the rest of the body. The visible part of the hair is called the shaft and is in fact dead tissue: the only living part of the hair is its root, the dermal papilla, which lies below the surface of the scalp in a depression known as the follicle. The dermal papilla is made up of cells that are fed by the bloodstream.

Each hair consists of three layers. The outer layer, or cuticle, is the hair's protective shield and has tiny overlapping scales. When the cuticle scales lie flat, the hair feels soft and looks glossy. If the cuticle scales have been damaged, the hair will be dull and brittle and will tangle easily.

Beneath the cuticle lies the cortex, which give hair strength and elasticity. The cortex also contains the pigment melanin, which gives hair its natural colour. At the centre of each hair is the

Below: Spring forward for great hair!

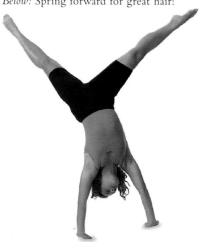

medulla, which is believed to supply the cortex and cuticle with nutrients.

Hair's natural shine is supplied by sebum, a conditioning oil composed of waxes and fats, which also contains a natural antiseptic to help fight infection. Sebum is produced by the sebaceous glands present in the dermis. The glands release sebum into the hair follicles. Sebum gives a protective coating to the hair shaft, smoothing the cuticle scales and helping hair retain moisture and elasticity. When the sebaceous glands produce too much sebum the result is greasy hair. Conversely, if too little sebum is produced the hair will be dry.

THE GROWTH CYCLE

The only living part of hair is underneath the scalp – when the hair has grown through the scalp it is dead tissue. There are three stages of hair growth: the anagen phase with active growth; the catagen, or transitional, phase when growth stops but cell activity continues; and the telogen phase, when all activity stops. When there is no further growth, the old hair is pushed out by the new growth and the cycle begins again.

Below: A sensible fitness plan means a boost to your health – and your hair.

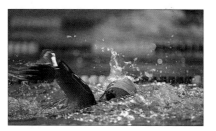

THE IMPORTANCE OF DIET

Like the rest of the body, healthy hair depends on a good diet to ensure it is supplied with all the nutrients it needs. However, if you eat a balanced diet with plenty of fresh ingredients you shouldn't need to take any supplementary vitamins to promote healthy hair growth.

An adequate supply of protein in the diet is essential to healthy hair. Good sources of protein include lean meat, poultry, fish, cheese and eggs as well as nuts, seeds and pulses. Fish, seaweed, nuts, yogurt and cottage cheese will all give hair strength and a natural shine. Wholegrain foods help in the formation of keratin, the major component of hair. Try to eat at least three pieces of fruit a day – it is packed with fibre, vitamins and minerals. Avoid saturated fat, which is found in red meat, fried foods and dairy products. Choose skimmed or semi-skimmed milk and low-fat cheese and yogurt, and substitute vegetable oils such as olive oil for animal fats.

Below: Silky hair is a real beauty asset!

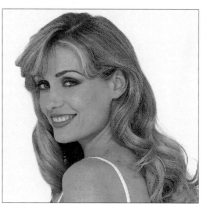

PROMOTING HEALTHY HAIR

■ Cut down on tea and coffee – they are powerful stimulants, increasing the excretion of water and nutrients and hampering the absorption of minerals. Drink between six and eight glasses of mineral water a day, along with herbal teas and unsweetened fruit juices.

■ Alcohol dilates blood vessels and increases blood flow to the tissues but is antagonistic to the nutrients vital for healthy hair, so limit yourself to an occasional drink.

■ Regular exercise stimulates the blood circulation, encouraging a supply of nutrients to the hair root.

Fact File

■ Hair grows about 1 cm/1/2 in per month.
■ A single strand of hair "lives" for up to seven years.
■ If a person never had their hair cut it would grow to a length of approximately 107 cm/42 in before falling out.
■ Women have more hair than men.
■ Hair grows faster in the summer months and during sleep.
■ Hair grows fastest between the ages of 16 and 24.

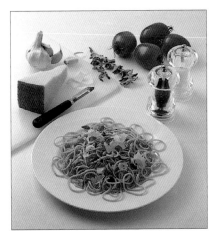

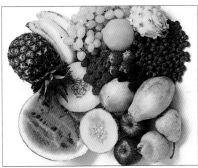

COLOUR

Hair colour is closely related to skin colour and is governed by the same pigment, melanin. The number of melanin granules in the cortex of the hair and the shape of the granules will determine a person's natural hair colour.

For most people the melanin granules are elongated in shape. People who have a large number of elongated melanin granules in the cortex have black hair, those with slightly fewer elongated granules have brown hair, and people with even less will be blonde. When the melanin granules are spherical or oval in shape the hair will appear red.

If spherical or oval granules appear in combination with a small number of elongated ones, then the hair will have rich, reddish-brown tinges. If spherical granules combine with a large number of elongated granules then the blackness of the hair will mask the redness, giving just a subtle tinge to the hair.

Hair colour darkens with age, but at some stage during middle-age the pigment formation slows down and silvery-grey hairs begin to appear. Gradually, the production of melanin ceases, and all the hair becomes colourless – or what is generally termed grey. When melanin granules are completely lacking from birth, as in albinos, the hair appears pure white.

Far left: Swap tea and coffee for healthy unsweetened fruit juices.

Above left: A balanced diet will supply all the nutrients you need for healthy hair.

Left: Eat lots of fresh fruit to help keep your hair shiny and soft.

Texture and Type

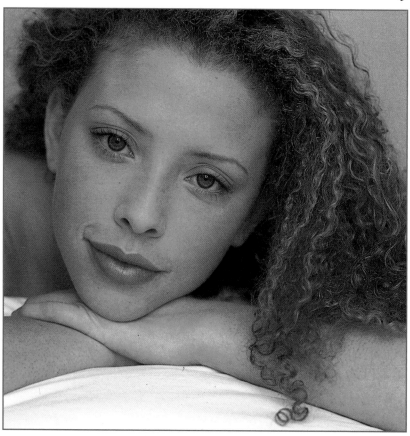

Fact File
■ Healthy hair is highly elastic and can stretch an extra 20 or 30 per cent of its length before snapping.
■ Chinese circus acrobats have been known to perform tricks while suspended by their hair.
■ A human hair is stronger than copper wire of the same thickness.
■ The combined strength of a headful of human hair is capable of supporting a weight equivalent to that of 99 people.

Left: Knowing your hair type is an important part of caring for your hair.

The texture of your hair is determined by the size and shape of the hair follicles, which is a genetic trait controlled by hormones and related to age and racial characteristics.

Whether hair is curly, wavy, or straight depends on two things: its shape as it grows out of the follicle and the distribution of keratin-producing cells at the roots. If viewed in cross-section, straight hair tends to be round, wavy hair tends to be oval, and curly hair kidney-shaped.

Straight hair is formed by roots that produce the same number of keratin cells around the follicle. In curly hair the production of keratin cells is uneven, so that there are more cells on one side of the oval-shaped follicle than on the other. Furthermore, the production of excess cells alternates between the sides, causing the developing hair to grow first in one direction and then in the other. The result of an imbalance in cell production will be curly hair.

The natural colour of the hair also affects the texture. Natural blondes have finer hair than brunettes while redheads have the thickest hair.

Hair can be divided into three categories: fine, medium, and coarse and thick. Fine hair can be strong or weak but, because of its texture, all fine hair lacks volume. Medium hair is neither thick nor thin and is strong and elastic. Thick and coarse hair is abundant and heavy, with a tendency to grow outwards from the scalp as well as downwards.

A single head of hair may consist of several different textures. Fine hair is found on the temples, hairline and at the nape of the head, while the texture over the rest of the head may be medium or even coarse.

DRY, NORMAL OR GREASY?

Hair type is determined by the amount of sebum the body produces. Treatment programmes such as perming, colouring, and heat styling will also have an effect on hair type, and sometimes the effects of these will be permanent. The different hair types are described below, together with advice on haircare.

Dry hair

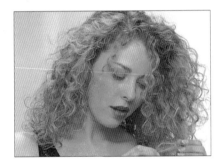

Hair that is too dry looks dull, feels dry, tangles easily and is difficult to comb or brush. It is often thick at the roots but thinner, and sometimes split, at the ends. **Causes** Excessive shampooing, overuse of heat-styling equipment, misuse of colour or perms, damage from the sun or harsh weather conditions. These factors deplete the moisture content of hair so that it loses its elasticity, bounce and suppleness. Dryness can also be the result of a sebum deficiency on the hair's surface, caused by a lack of or decrease in sebaceous gland secretions. **Solutions** Use a nourishing shampoo and an intensive conditioner specifically for dry hair. Treat the hair as gently as you can: allow hair to dry naturally whenever possible. Consider having a trim if you have split ends.

Normal hair

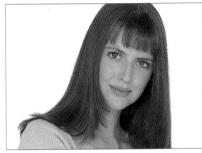

Normal hair is neither greasy nor dry, has not been permed or coloured, holds its style and looks good most of the time.

Greasy hair

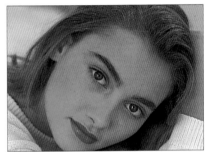

This looks lank and oily and is often unmanageable. It needs frequent washing. **Causes** Overproduction of sebum as a result of hormone disturbances, stress, excessive brushing, perspiration or a diet rich in saturated fat. **Solutions** Use a gentle shampoo that also gives the hair volume. A light perm will lift the hair at the roots and limit the dispersal of sebum. Rethink your diet: reduce dairy fats and greasy foods. Eat plenty of fresh foods, and drink six to eight glasses of water every day.

Combination hair

Combination hair is greasy at the roots but dry and sometimes split at the ends. **Causes** Chemical treatments, overuse of detergent-based shampoos, overexposure to sunlight and overuse of heat styling equipment. Repeated abuse provokes a reaction in sebum secretion at the roots and an alteration in the scales, which can no longer fulfil their protective role. As a result, the hair ends become dry. **Solutions** Use only gentle products on the hair. Formulations for oily hair and for dry hair may contribute to the problem, so use a product designed for combination hair. If this is not possible try using a shampoo for oily hair and finish by applying a conditioner only from the middle lengths to the ends of the hair.

Coloured or permed hair

Hair that has been coloured or permed is often more porous than untreated hair and needs careful handling, using gentle cleansers and quality conditioners. Colour-care products help to prevent fading by protecting the hair from sunlight. Specialist products for permed hair help maintain elasticity.

Below: Clever haircare means great hair.

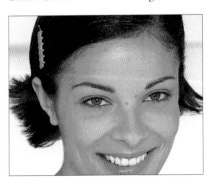

The Cut

Hair growth varies over different parts of the head. This is why your cut can appear to be out of shape very quickly.

As a general rule, a short precision cut needs trimming every four weeks, a longer style every six to eight weeks.

Even if you want to grow your hair you should have it trimmed at least every three months to prevent splitting.

Hairdressers use a variety of techniques and tools to make hair appear thicker, fuller, straighter or curlier, according to the desired effect. The techniques and tools they use are explained below.

Blunt cutting

This is when the ends are cut straight across; it is often used for hair of one length and for fine hair. The weight and fullness of the hair is distributed around the perimeter of the shape.

Clippers

Clippers are used for close-cut styles and sometimes to finish off a cut. Shaved clipper cuts need to be trimmed very regularly to keep the style.

Graduated hair

Graduated hair is cut at an angle to give lots of fullness on top and to gradually blend the top hair into shorter lengths at the nape.

Layering

Layering the hair evenly distributes the weight and fullness, giving a soft and round appearance to the style.

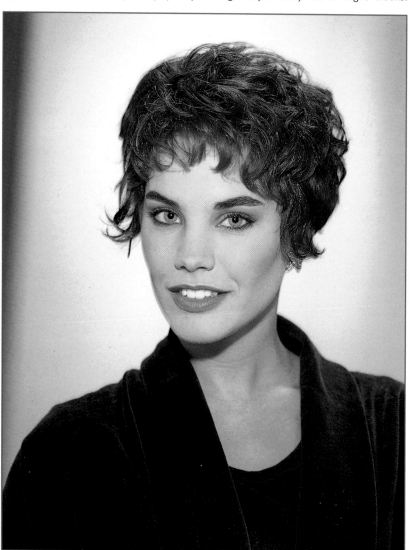

Left: This permed style was cut into a short crop with heavy layers. The hair was diffuser-dried to give extra movement, then sculpting gel was used to emphasize the side kicks and styling lotion was added for a textured look.

Slide cutting

This technique (also called slithering or feathering) thins the hair. Scissors are used in a sliding action, backwards and forwards along the hair length, often when the hair is dry.

Razor cutting

Razor cutting creates softness, tapering and internal movement so that the hair moves more freely. It can also be used to shorten hair. Thinning hair, either with thinning scissors or a razor, removes bulk and weight without affecting the overall length of the hair.

CLEVER CUTS

■ Fine, thin, flyaway hair can be given extra volume and movement by blunt cutting. Mid-length hair can be given volume, while short, thin hair can have the edges graduated to give movement.

■ Fine hair can also be razor cut for a thicker and more voluminous effect. Do not let fine hair grow long. As soon as it reaches the shoulders it can look wispy.

■ Thick hair can be controlled by reducing the weight to give more style and direction. Avoid very short styles because the hair will tend to stick out. Try a layered cut with added movement.

■ Layering the hair also helps achieve height and eliminate weight. On shorter styles the weight can be reduced with thinning scissors used on the ends only.

■ Hair can grow in different directions, causing styling problems. For example, a cowlick is normally found on the front hairline and occurs when the hair grows

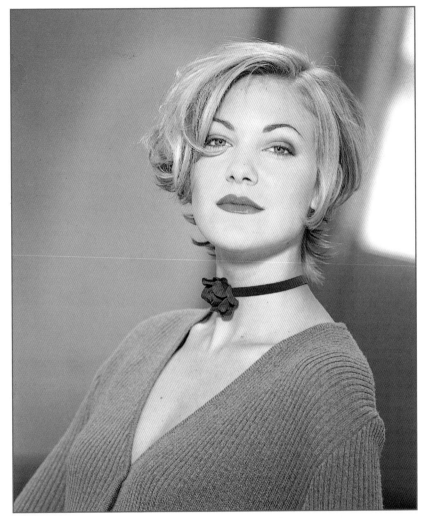

in a swirl, backwards and then forwards. Clever cutting can redistribute the weight and go some way towards solving the problem. For a double crown – when there are two pivots of hair, rather than the usual one – choose a style which gives height at the crown.

Above: For this sleek seventies look, extra body was given to fine hair with a razor cut to create movement. The hair was blow-dried using a large round brush to pull the hair straight. Finally, sculpting wax was used to give maximum smoothness and shine.

Shampoo Success

Shampoos are designed to cleanse the hair and scalp, removing dirt and grime without stripping away too much of the natural sebum. They contain cleansing agents, perfume, preservatives and conditioning agents that can coat the hair shaft to make the hair appear thicker. The conditioning agents smooth the cuticle scales so the hair doesn't tangle and help to eliminate static electricity from the hair when it dries.

THE pH FACTOR

The letters pH refer to the acid/alkaline level of a substance. It is calculated on a scale of 1 to 14. Numbers below 7 denote acidity, those over 7 alkalinity. Most shampoos range between a pH factor of 5 and 7; medicated varieties have a pH of about 7.3, which is near neutral. Sebum has a pH factor of between 4.5 and 5.5, which is mildly acidic. Bacteria cannot survive in this pH, and maintaining this protective layer keeps the scalp and hair at their best.

Below: Choose your shampoo carefully.

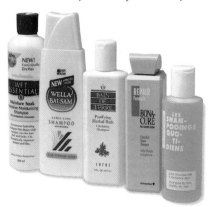

SHAMPOO TIPS

■ Always use the correct shampoo for your hair type.

■ Don't wash your hair in washing-up liquid or soap; they are highly alkaline and will upset your hair's natural pH balance by stripping out the natural oils.

■ Always read the instructions first: some shampoos need to be left on the scalp for a few minutes before rinsing.

■ Buy small sachets of shampoo to test which brand is most suitable for you.

■ Don't wash your hair in the bath; dirty bath water is not conducive to clean hair, and it is difficult to rinse properly without a shower attachment or separate jug.

■ Always wash your brush and comb when you shampoo your hair.

■ Change your shampoo approximately every two weeks; hair develops a resistance to certain ingredients after time.

■ Don't throw away a shampoo that doesn't lather. The amount of suds are determined by the active level of detergent, as well as by the hardness of the water in your area.

■ Many shampoos are labelled "pH balanced", and this means they have the same acidity level as hair. Use a shampoo of this type if you have permed or coloured hair. These shampoos are not necessary for normal hair, as long as you condition your hair after shampooing.

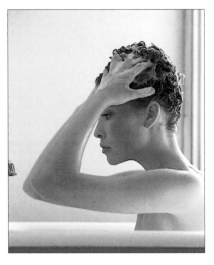

Above: If you wash your hair regularly use a mild shampoo.

Below: Rinse your hair with warm water after shampooing. Continue to rinse until the water runs clear and clean.

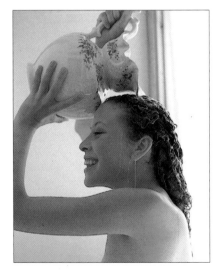

GETTING IT RIGHT

■ Always use a product formulated for your particular hair type, and before shampooing brush your hair to free any tangles and loosen dirt and dead skin cells.

■ Use lukewarm water, as hot water can be uncomfortable on the scalp. Wet the hair, then apply a small amount of shampoo and massage into the roots, using the pads of your fingertips; never use your nails. Pay attention to the hairline area, where make-up and dirt become trapped. Don't rub vigorously or you will stretch the hair.

■ After shampooing, rinse thoroughly until the water runs clean and clear. Repeat only if you think your hair needs it. Blot the hair with a clean towel to remove excess water.

MASSAGING THE SCALP

Massage helps maintain a healthy scalp by improving the circulation and delivering nutrients and oxygen to the hair follicle. It also helps loosen dead skin cells and can redress the overproduction of sebum, which makes hair greasy.

You can give yourself a scalp massage at home. Use warm olive oil if the scalp is dry or tight. Try equal parts of witch hazel and mineral water if you have an oily scalp. For a normal scalp, use equal parts rose and mineral waters.

■ Begin the massage by gently rotating your scalp using the tips of your fingers, taking care not to use your nails. Start the massage at the forehead, move across to the sides and then work over the crown to the nape of the neck. Try to keep the movement continuous.

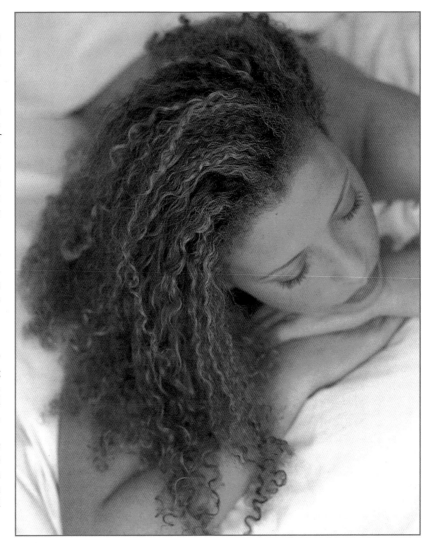

■ Next, place your fingertips firmly on your scalp without exerting too much pressure. Push your fingers together, then pull them apart through the hair in a gentle kneading motion, without lifting or moving them.

■ Massage for a minute, then move to the next section. Treat your entire scalp and upper neck in this way.

Above: Healthy, shiny hair looks great and reflects good physical well-being.

Getting into Condition

Few people are able to wash their hair and let the matter rest at that; most need help just to overcome the effects of modern living, not to mention the occasional problem that needs treatment. Here is a guide to the range of products available to get hair back into condition.

THE CONDITIONERS

Glossy hair has cuticle scales that lie flat and neatly overlap, reflecting the light. Perming and colouring, rough handling and heat styling all conspire to lift the cuticles, allowing moisture to be lost from the cortex and making hair dry, lacklustre, and prone to tangles. Severely damaged cuticles break off completely, which means that the hair gets thinner and eventually breaks.

To put the shine back into hair it may be necessary to use a specific conditioner that meets the hair's requirements. Conditioners, with the exception of hot oils, should be applied to freshly shampooed hair that has first been blotted dry with a clean towel to remove the excess moisture.

Basic conditioners

These coat the hair with a fine film, temporarily smoothing down the cuticle and making the hair glossier and easier to manage. Leave for a few minutes before rinsing thoroughly.

Conditioning sprays

These are used prior to styling and form a protective barrier against the harmful effects of heat. They are also good for reducing static electricity on flyaway hair.

Hot oils

These give an intensive, deep nourishing treatment. To use, place the unopened tube in a cup of hot water and leave for one minute. Wet the hair and towel it dry. Massage the hot oil evenly into the scalp and hair. For a more intensive treatment, cover the head with a shower cap. To finish, rinse the hair and shampoo.

Intensive conditioners

These help hair to replenish its natural moisture balance. Use this type if the hair is split, dry, frizzy or difficult to manage. Distribute the conditioner through the hair and allow it to penetrate for two to five minutes. Rinse well with fresh water, lifting your hair from the scalp to wash away any residue.

Below: Condition when and where your hair needs it, not just for the sake of it.

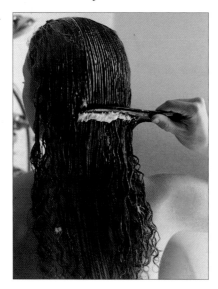

Leave-in conditioners

These are designed to help retain moisture, reduce static and add shine. They are especially good for fine hair as they avoid conditioner overload, which can cause lankness. Convenient and easy-to-use, they also provide a protective barrier against the effects of heat styling. Apply after shampooing but don't rinse off. These products are ideal for daily use.

Restructurants

Restructurants penetrate the cortex, helping to repair and strengthen the inner part of damaged hair. They are helpful if the hair is lank and limp and has lost its natural elasticity as a result of chemical treatments or physical damage.

Split end treatments/serums

Split end treatments and serums condition damaged hair. The best course of action for split ends is to have the ends trimmed, but this does not always solve the whole problem because the hair tends to break off and split at different levels. As an intermediate solution, split ends can be temporarily sealed using specialist conditioners. They are worked into the ends of newly washed hair so that they surround the hair with a microscopic film that leaves the hair shaft smoother.

Colour/perm conditioners

Conditioners for coloured or permed hair are specially designed for chemically treated hair. After-colour products add a protective film around porous areas of the hair, preventing colour loss. After-perm products help stabilize the hair and help to keep the bounce in the curl.

PROBLEMS AND SOLUTIONS

The following hair problems are easily overcome with an appropriate treatment.

Dandruff

Dandruff consists of scaly particles with an oily sheen that lie close to the root.
Causes Poor diet, sluggish metabolism, stress, hormonal imbalance or infection can all increase cell renewal on the scalp, meaning an increase in sebum. The scales will absorb some of the excess oil, but the problem will worsen unless treated.
Solutions Brush the hair before shampooing, using a mild anti-dandruff shampoo to loosen the scales. Follow with a treatment lotion. Avoid excessive use of heat stylers. If the problem persists, consult your family doctor.

Flaky/itchy scalp

This produces tiny pieces of dead skin that flake off the scalp. The scalp can be red or itchy, and the hair looks dull.

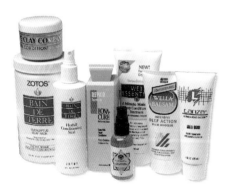

Above: The range of conditioning products now available means that hair problems can be a thing of the past.

Causes Hereditary traits, stress, shampoo residues caused by insufficient rinsing, lack of sebum, harsh shampoos, air conditioning, pollution and central heating.
Solutions Choose a moisturizing shampoo and use a conditioner with herbal extracts to help soothe the scalp.

Fine hair

Fine hair tends to be limp, looks flat and does not hold a style.
Causes The texture is hereditary, but the problem is often made worse by using too heavy a conditioner, which weighs the hair down. Excessive use of styling products can have the same effect.
Solutions Wash the hair with a mild shampoo and use a light conditioner. Volumizing shampoos can help give body, and soft perms will make the hair appear thicker and the style fuller.

Frizzy hair

Frizzy hair results from air moisture being absorbed into the hair. The hair looks dry and lacklustre, and is difficult to control.
Causes Can be inherited or caused by rough treatment, such as too much harsh brushing or pulling the hair into bands.
Solutions When washing the hair, massage the shampoo into the roots and allow the lather to work to the ends. Apply a conditioner from the mid-length of the hair to the ends, or use a leave-in conditioner. The hair is best styled with gel, applied when the hair is wet. The hair can also be dried naturally.

Split ends

Split ends occur when the cuticle is damaged and the fibres of the cortex unravel. The hair is dry, brittle and prone to tangling and can be split at the end.

Causes Over-perming or colouring, insufficient conditioning or too much brushing or backcombing. Careless use of rollers and hairpins, excessive heat styling and not having a regular trim.
Solutions Split ends can't be mended; the only long-term cure is to have them snipped off. What is lost in the length will be gained in quality. Shampoo less often and never use a dryer too near the hair or set it on too high a temperature. Try conditioners and serums that are designed to temporarily seal split ends and give resistance to further splitting.

Product build-up

This is the residue of styling products left on the hair shaft.
Causes Residues combine with mineral deposits in the water and a build-up occurs. The hair is difficult to perm or colour because of a barrier preventing the chemicals from penetrating the hair.
Solutions Use a stripping or clarifying shampoo specially designed to remove product build-up. This is particularly important prior to perming or colouring.

Below: Your hair needs careful handling if it is to look its best!

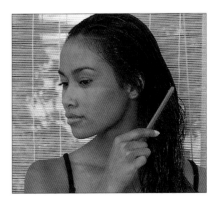

Colouring and Bleaching

Hair colourants have never been better than those available today; nowadays it is a simple matter to add a temporary tone and gloss to the hair or even to make a more permanent change. And there is a wide choice of home colouring products if you like the idea of experimenting yourself.

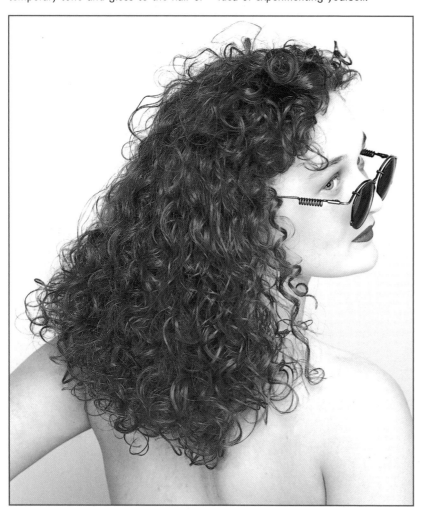

Above: Adding colour to your hair swells the hair and makes it look thicker, and this in turn adds texture and gives the appearance of a healthy head of hair.

THE CHOICE

There is a wide range of colouring products available and it helps to know what is on offer before you decide.

Temporary colours

These are usually water-based and are applied to pre-shampooed, wet hair. They work by coating the outside, or cuticle layer, of the hair. The colour washes away in the next shampoo.

Colour setting

Colour setting lotions combine a colour that washes out with a strong setting lotion. They are similar to temporary colours and are perfect for adding tone to grey, white or bleached hair.

Semi-permanent colours

These give a more noticeable effect that lasts for six to eight shampoos. They can only add, enrich, or darken hair colour, they cannot make it any lighter. These colours penetrate the cuticle and coat the outer edge of the cortex. The colour fades gradually and is ideal for those who just want to experiment. Longer lasting semi-permanent colours remain in the hair for 12–20 shampoos. The colour penetrates deeper into the cortex than in semi-permanent colour. This type is perfect for a more lasting change.

Permanent colours

These can be used to lighten or darken hair permanently. The colour is absorbed by the cortex in around 30 minutes, and after this time oxygen in the developer swells the pigments in the colourant and holds them in. The roots may need retouching every six weeks. When retouching it is important to colour only the new hair growth. If the new colour overlaps previously treated hair there will be a build-up of colour from the mid-lengths to the ends, which will make the hair more porous.

NATURAL COLOURING

Vegetable colourants such as henna and chamomile have been used since ancient times to colour hair. Henna is the most widely used natural dye, but colourants can be extracted from a wide variety of plants, including marigold petals, cloves, rhubarb stalks and even tea leaves.

Natural dyes work in the same way as semi-permanent colourants by staining the outside of the hair. However, results are variable and a residue is often left behind, making further colouring with permanent tints or bleaches inadvisable.

Right: Gentle natural colourants, containing herbs and minerals, are available for adding tone and shine.

Henna

Henna enhances natural highlights and makes colour appear richer. The colour fades gradually but frequent applications will give a stronger, longer-lasting effect.

The result that is achieved when using henna depends on the natural colour of the hair. On brunette or black hair it produces a lovely reddish glow, while lighter hair becomes a beautiful titian. Henna is not suitable for use on blonde hair, and on hair that is more than 20 per cent tinted, bleached or highlighted, the resultant colour will be orange.

Always test the henna you intend to use on a few loose hairs (the ones in your hairbrush will do), making a note of the length of time it takes to produce the result you want.

Use neutral henna to add gloss without adding colour. Mix henna and water to a stiff paste. Stir in an egg yolk and a little milk, and mix. Apply to the hair and leave for an hour before rinsing. Repeat every two months.

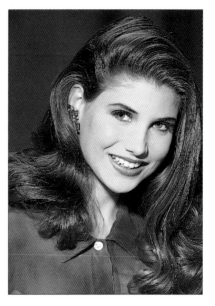

Above: Colour-treated hair needs extra care if it is to really shine! Pay close attention to the look and feel of your hair so that you can be ready to respond straight away if problems occur.

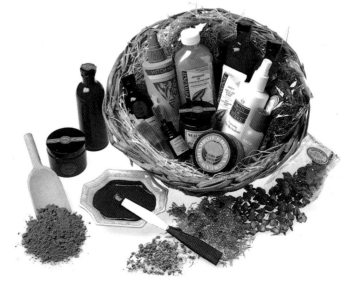

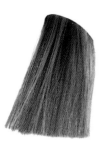

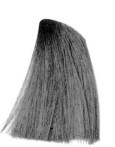

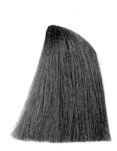

DO'S AND DON'TS

■ Do rinse henna paste thoroughly or the hair and scalp will feel gritty.

■ Don't expose hennaed hair to strong sunlight, and rinse salt and chlorine from the hair immediately after swimming.

■ Do use a henna shampoo between colour applications to enhance the tone.

■ Don't use shampoos and conditioners containing henna on blonde, grey or chemically treated hair.

■ Do use the same henna product each time you apply henna.

■ Don't use compound henna (with added metallic salts); it can cause long-term hair colouring problems.

Chamomile

Chamomile has a gentle lightening effect on hair and is good for sun-streaking blonde and light brown hair. However, it takes several applications and a good deal of time to produce the desired effect. The advantage of chamomile over chemical bleach is that it never gives a brassy or yellow tone.

To make a chamomile rinse to use after each shampoo, place 30 ml/2 tbsp dried chamomile flowers in 600 ml/ 1 pint boiling water. Simmer for about 15 minutes, strain and cool before use.

For a stronger rinse, add 125 g/1 cup dried chamomile flowers to 300 ml/ ½ pint boiling water and leave to steep for 15 minutes. Cool, simmer, and strain. Add the juice of a lemon plus 30 ml/ 2 tbsp rich cream conditioner. Comb through the hair and leave to dry – in the sun, if possible. Finally, shampoo and condition your hair as usual.

CHOOSING A NEW COLOUR

When choosing a colour a basic rule is to keep to one or two shades at each side of your original tone. It is best to try a temporary colourant first; if you like the result you can choose a semi-permanent or permanent colourant next time. If you want to be a platinum blonde and you are a natural brunette, you should seek the advice of a professional hairdresser.

There are two points to remember when considering a colour change. First, only have a colour change if your hair is in good condition; dry, porous hair absorbs colour too rapidly, leading to a patchy result. Second, your make-up may need changing to suit your new colour.

SPECIAL TECHNIQUES

Hairdressers over the years have devised colouring methods and techniques to create different effects. These are some of the choices available.

Flying colours

A combination of colours is applied with combs and brushes to the middle lengths and tips of the hair.

Highlights/lowlights

Fine strands of hair are tinted or bleached lighter or darker, or colour is added to give varying colour tones throughout the hair and to give the appearance of depth and texture. This technique can be called frosting or shimmering, particularly when bleach is used to give an overall lighter effect.

Slices

In this technique assorted colours are applied throughout the hair to emphasize the cut and to show movement.

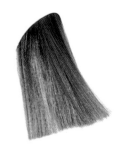

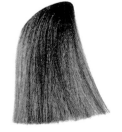

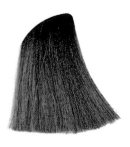

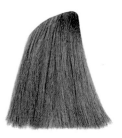

COVERING WHITE HAIR

To cover a few white hairs, use a temporary or semi-permanent colour that will last for six to eight weeks. Choose one that is similar to your natural colour. If the hair is brown, applying a warm brown colour will pick out the white areas and give lighter chestnut highlights. Alternatively, henna will give a glossy finish and produce stunning red highlights. For salt and pepper hair – hair with a mixed amount of white with the natural colour – try a longer lasting semi-permanent colour. These last for up to 20 shampoos and will also add shine.

When hair is completely white it can be covered with a permanent tint, but it will be necessary to update the colour every four to six weeks. You can enhance your natural shade of white by using toning shampoos, conditioners and styling products to remove brassiness and add some beautiful silvery tones.

CARING FOR COLOURED HAIR

Chlorinated and salt water, perspiration and the weather can all fade coloured hair, particularly hair that has been coloured red. Specialist products are available to help counteract fading, such as those with ultraviolet filters to protect coloured hair from the damaging effects of the sun's rays. Always rinse your hair thoroughly in chlorine-free water after swimming and use a shampoo designed for coloured hair, followed by a separate conditioner. Gently blot the hair after shampooing – never rub it vigorously as this ruffles the cuticle and can result in colour "escaping". It is a good idea to use an intensive conditioning treatment at least once a month to help prolong the colourant.

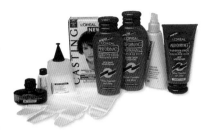

Above: Specially formulated care products.

BLEACHING

Bleaching gives a change in hair colour by removing colour from the hair. There are several different types of bleach available, ranging from mild brighteners that lift hair colour a couple of shades to more powerful mixes that completely strip hair of its natural colour.

Bleaching is difficult to do and is best left to a professional hairdresser. If misused it can be harsh and drying on the hair. For best results make sure your hair is in optimum condition before bleaching, and regularly apply an intensive conditioner to your hair afterwards.

COLOUR CORRECTION

If you have coloured your hair and want to go back to your natural colour without waiting for the colour to grow out, consult a professional hairdresser. Hair that has been tinted darker than its normal shade will have to be colour-stripped with a bleach bath until the desired colour is achieved. Hair that has been bleached or highlighted will need to be re-pigmented and then tinted to match the original colour. For best results, these processes should be carried out in a salon, using specialist products.

HELPFUL HINTS FOR HOME HAIR COLOURING

■ Always read the directions supplied with the product before you start, and follow them precisely. Make sure you first do a strand and skin sensitivity test.

■ If retouching the roots of tinted or bleached hair, apply new colour only to the regrowth area. Any overlap will result in uneven colour and porosity, which will affect the condition of your hair.

■ Don't colour your hair at home if the hair is split or visibly damaged, or if you have used bleach or henna; always allow previously treated hair to grow out first.

■ Avoid colouring your hair if taking prescribed drugs, as the chemical balance of your hair can alter. Check with your family doctor first.

■ If your hair has been permed, consult a hairdresser before using a hair colourant. If you are in any doubt about using a colour, check with the manufacturer or consult a professional hair colourist.

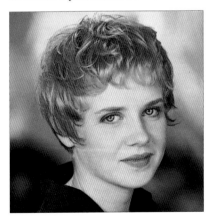

Above: A change of colour can give an instant lift to your hairstyle.

Permanent Solutions

Making straight hair curly is not a new idea. Women in ancient Egypt coated their hair in mud, wound it around wooden rods and then used the heat from the sun to create the curls. Waves that won't wash out are a more recent innovation. Improved formulations and sophisticated techniques have made perms the most versatile styling option in hairdressing.

How they Work

Perms work by breaking down the inner structures (links) in your hair and reforming them to give a new shape. A perming lotion alters the keratin and breaks down the sulphur bonds that link the fibre-like cells together in the inner layers of the hair. When the fibres are loose, the hair is stretched over a curler or a perming rod to give a new shape.

Once the curlers or rods are in place, more lotion is applied and the perm is left to fix the new shape. The development time varies according to the condition and texture of the hair. When the development is complete, the changed links in the hair are re-formed into their new shape by the application of a neutralizer. The neutralizer contains an oxidizing agent that is responsible for closing up the broken links and producing the wave or curl – permanently.

The type of curl that is produced depends on the size of the curler. Generally speaking, the smaller the curler the smaller and tighter the curl, whereas medium to large curlers tend to give a much looser effect. The strength of the lotion and the type and texture of the hair can also make a difference.

Home versus Salon

Perming is a delicate operation, and it is often a good idea to leave it to trained and experienced professional hairdressers. The advantages of having hair permed in a salon are several. The hair is first analyzed to see whether it is in fit condition to take a perm; coloured, out-of-condition or over-processed hair may not be suitable and you will be then given specific advice on how to get your hair back into shape. A professional perm also offers more choice in the type of curl available – different strengths of lotion and different winding techniques all give a wider range of curls, many of which are not available in home perms.

Post Perm Tips

■ Don't wash newly permed hair for 48 hours after processing as any stress can cause curls to relax.
■ Use shampoos and conditioners formulated for permed hair to help retain the correct moisture balance and prolong the perm.
■ Always use a wide-toothed comb and work from the ends upwards. Never brush the hair.
■ Blot wet hair dry before styling to prevent stretching.
■ Avoid using too much heat on permed hair. If possible, wash, condition and let dry naturally.
■ If your perm has lost its bounce, mist with water or try a curl reviver. These are designed to put instant volume and bounce into permed hair.

Don't do it yourself if . . .

■ Your hair is very dry or damaged.

■ You have bleached or highlighted your hair: it may be too fragile. If in doubt, check with your hairdresser.

■ The traces of an old perm still remain in your hair.

■ You suffer from a scalp disorder such as eczema or have broken, irritated skin.

Below: Spiral perming gives a ringlet effect on long hair.

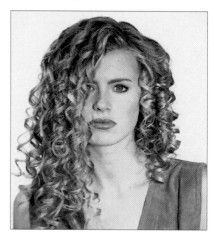

Salon Perms – The Choices

Professional hairdressers usually offer a number of different types of perm that are not available for home use.

Acid perms

These produce highly conditioned, flexible curls. They are ideally suited to hair that is fine, sensitive, fragile, damaged, or tinted, as they have a mildly acidic action that minimizes the risk of hair damage.

Alkaline perms

Alkaline perms give strong, firm curl results on normal and resistant hair.

Exothermic perms

These give bouncy, resilient curls. "Exothermic" refers to the gentle heat that is produced by the chemical reaction that occurs when the lotion is mixed. The heat allows the lotion to penetrate the hair cuticle, strengthening the hair as the hair moulds into its new shape.

PERMING TECHNIQUES

Any of the above types of perm can be used with different techniques to produce a number of results.

Body perms

These are soft, loose perms created by using large curlers, or sometimes rollers. The result is added volume with a hint of wave and movement rather than curls.

Root perms

To add lift and volume in the root area only. They are ideal for fine or short hair that tends to go flat.

Pin curl perms

These give soft, natural waves and curls, which are achieved by perming small sections of hair that have been pinned into pre-formed curls.

Stack perms

A stack perm gives curl and volume to one-length haircuts by means of different sized curlers. The hair on top of the head is left unpermed while the middle and ends have more curl and movement. The hair should be cut before the perm is applied.

Spiral perms

These create spiral curls by winding the hair around special curlers. The mass of curls makes long hair look much thicker.

Spot perms

Spot perms give support only on the area to which they are applied. If the hair needs lift the perm is applied just on the crown. They can also be used on the fringe (bangs) or on areas around the face.

Weave perms

Sections of hair are permed while the rest of the hair is left straight to give a mixture of texture and natural looking body and bounce, particularly on areas around the face.

REGROWTH PROBLEM

When a perm is growing out, the areas of new growth should only be permed if a barrier is created between old and new growth. The barrier can be a special cream or a plastic protector, both of which effectively prevent the perming lotion and neutralizer from touching previously permed areas.

Specially formulated products for re-perming a length of hair without damaging its structure are available from professional salons.

Below: Give thick hair a volume perm to produce a beautiful abundance of curls and the fullest look possible.

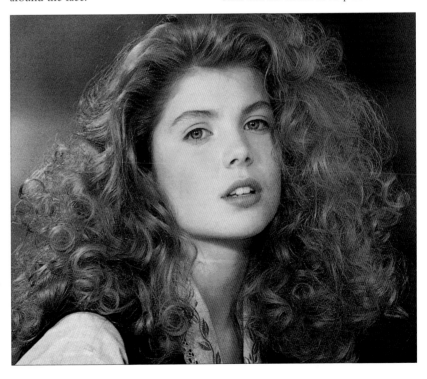

A Style to Suit your Face

Make the most of your looks by choosing a style that maximizes your best features. The first feature you should consider is your face shape – is it round, oval, square or long? If you are not sure what shape it is scrape your hair back off your face. Stand squarely in front of a mirror and use a lipstick to trace the outline of your face on to the mirror. When you stand back you should be able to see into which of the following categories your face shape falls.

THE SQUARE FACE

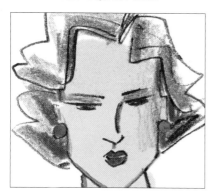

The square face is angular with a broad forehead and a square jawline. To make the best of this shape, choose a hairstyle with long layers, preferably one with soft waves or curls, as these create a softness that detracts from the hard lines. Part the hair on the side of the head and comb the fringe away from the face.
Styles to avoid: Severe geometric cuts – they will only emphasize squareness; long bobs with heavy fringes; severe styles in which the hair is scraped off the face and parted down the centre.

THE ROUND FACE

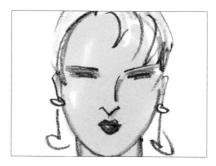

On the round face the distance between the forehead and the chin is about equal to the distance between the cheeks. Choose a style with a short fringe, which lengthens the face, and a short cut, which makes the face look thinner.
Styles to avoid: Curly styles, because they emphasize the roundness; very full, long hair or severe styles.

THE OVAL FACE

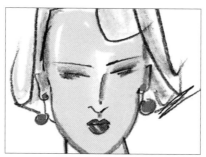

The oval face has wide cheekbones that taper down into a small chin and up to a narrow forehead. This is regarded as the perfect face shape and has the advantage of being able to wear any hairstyle well.

THE LONG FACE

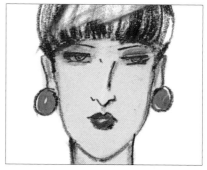

The long face has a high forehead and long chin and needs to be given the illusion of width. Soften the effect with short layers, or go for a bob with a fringe, to create horizontal lines. Curly or scrunch-dried bobs balance out a long face very well.
Styles to avoid: Styles without fringes, and long, straight, one-length cuts.

The Complete You
A hairstyle affects your whole apperance, not just that of your face. When choosing a new hairstyle you should take into account your overall body shape. If you are a traditional pear-shape don't choose an elfin hairstyle; it will draw attention to the lower half of your body, making your hips look wide. Petite women should avoid masses of very curly hair as this makes the head appear out of proportion with the rest of the body.

If You Wear Glasses . . .

Try to choose frames and a hairstyle that complement each other. Large spectacles could spoil a neat, feathery cut, and very fine frames could be overpowered by a large, voluminous style. Remember to take your glasses to the salon when having your hair restyled so that your stylist can take their shape into consideration when deciding on the overall effect.

SPECIFIC PROBLEMS

■ Prominent nose: choose a hairstyle that incorporates softness into your appearance. A wispy fringe would work well, and a light perm would add height and movement, to balance out your face.

■ Pointed chin: you need to style your hair with plenty of width at the jawline. Don't have your hair cut too short.

■ Low forehead: choose a style with a wispy fringe, rather than one with a full fringe. Choose softer styles and avoid anything too severe.

■ High forehead: this is best disguised with a mid-length fringe.

■ Receding chin: select a hairstyle that comes just below chin level, ideally with lots of waves or curls around your shoulders.

■ Uneven hairline: a fringe should easily manage to conceal this problem.

Right: Your hairstyle has a big influence on your appearance, so be honest with yourself and take a critical look in the mirror before choosing a new style.

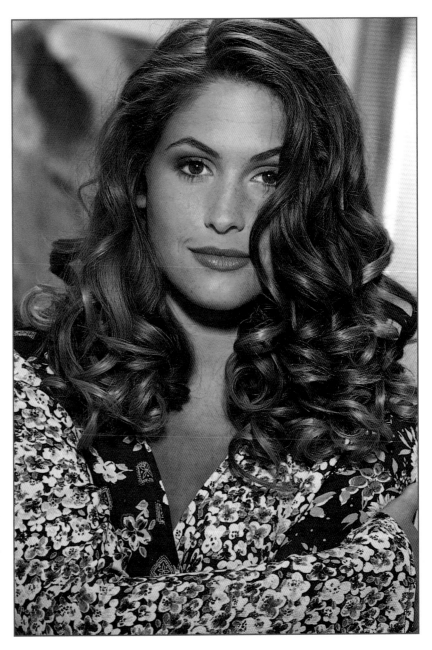

Styling Tools

The right tools not only make hair-styling more fun, but also make it much easier. Brushes, combs and pins are the basic tools of styling. The following is a guide to help you choose what is most suitable from the wide range that is available.

BRUSHES

Brushes are made of bristles, which may be natural hog bristle, plastic, nylon or wire. The bristles are embedded in a wooden, plastic or moulded rubber base and set in tufts or rows. This allows loose hair to collect in the grooves without interfering with the action of the bristles. The spacing of the tufts plays an important role – generally, the wider the spacing between the rows the easier the brush will flow through the hair.

The role of brushing

Brushes help to remove tangles and knots and smooth the hair. The action of brushing from the roots to the ends removes dead skin cells and dirt and encourages the cuticles to lie flat, reflecting the light. Brushing also stimulates the circulation, promoting hair growth.

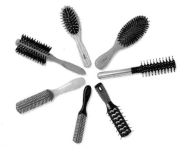

Above: Brushes should be carefully chosen and well looked after.

> **Tip**
> Replace brushes and combs with damaged bristles or broken teeth; the sharp edges can damage your scalp. Keep your brushes and combs to yourself, never lend to other people.

Cleaning

All brushes should be cleaned, at least once a week, by pulling out dead hairs and washing in warm, soapy water, then rinsing thoroughly. Natural bristle brushes should be left to dry naturally. If you use a pneumatic brush with a rubber cushion base, block the air hole with a matchstick before washing.

Plastic, nylon or wire bristles

All of these bristles are easily cleaned and are heat resistant, so they are good for blow-drying. They are available in a variety of shapes and styles. Cushioned brushes give good flexibility as they glide through the hair, preventing tugging and helping to remove knots. They are also non-static. A major disadvantage is that the ends can be harsh, so try to choose bristles with rounded or ball tips.

TYPES OF BRUSH

Circular or radial brushes

These brushes come in a variety of sizes and are circular or semicircular in shape. Circular or radial brushes have either mixed bristles for finishing a style, a rubber pad with nylon bristles for general use or metal pins specifically for styling. They are used to control naturally curly, permed and wavy hair and are ideal for blow-drying.

Flat or half-round brushes

These are ideal for wet or dry hairstyling and blow-drying. Normally they are made of nylon bristles in a rubber base.

Pneumatic brushes

These brushes have a domed rubber base with bristles set in tufts. They can be plastic, natural bristle or both.

Vent brushes

Vent brushes have hollow centres and special bristle, or pin, patterns that are designed to lift and disentangle hair. The air circulates freely through both the brush and the hair so the hair dries faster.

COMBS

Good quality combs have saw-cut teeth: each individual tooth is cut into the comb, so there are no sharp edges. Avoid cheap plastic combs that are made in a mould and form lines down the centre of the teeth. These scrape away the cuticle layers of the hair, eventually causing damage. Use a wide-toothed comb for disentangling and combing conditioner through the hair. Fine tail combs are for styling; Afro combs are for curly hair; and styling combs are for grooming.

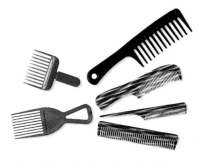

Above: Your choice of comb will vary according to the texture of your hair.

PINS AND CLIPS

These are indispensable for sectioning and securing hair during setting and for putting hair up. Most pins are available with untipped, plain ends, or cushion tipped ends. Non-reflective finishes are available, so the pins are less noticeable in the hair, and most are made of metal, plastic or stainless steel. Colours and styles vary from plain to adorned and highly decorative fashion accessories.

Double-pronged clips

These are most frequently used for making pin or barrel curls. Grips on the clips give added security to all types of curls, French pleats and the most intricately upswept styles.

Heavy hairpins

These are made of strong metal and come either waved or straight. They are ideal for securing rollers or for putting hair up.

Fine hairpins

These are used for dressing hair. They are delicate and prone to bend out of shape, so they should only be used to secure small amounts of hair. Fine hairpins are easily concealed, especially if you use a matching colour. They are sometimes used to secure pin curls during setting as heavier clips can leave a mark.

Sectioning clips

These clips have a single prong. They are often used to hold hair while working on another section, or securing pin curls.

Twisted pins

These are fashioned like a screw and are used to secure hairstyles such as chignons and French pleats.

ROLLERS

Rollers vary in diameter, length and the material from which they are made. Smooth rollers – those without spikes or brushes – will give the sleekest finish, but can be difficult to put in. More popular are brush rollers, especially the self-fixing variety that do not need pins or clips.

> **Tip**
> The smaller the roller, the tighter the curl. Keep the tension even when winding and do not buckle the ends of the hair.

SHAPERS

Shapers were inspired by the principle of rag-rolling hair and are a natural way to curl hair. Soft "twist tie" shapers are made from pliable rubber, plastic or cotton, with a tempered wire in the centre to enable it to bend into shape. The waves or curls that are produced are soft and bouncy and the technique is gentle enough for permed or tinted hair.

To use, section clean, dry hair and pull to a firm tension, "trapping" the end in a shaper that you have previously doubled over. Roll down to the roots and fold over to secure. Leave for 30–60 minutes without heat. For a more voluminous style, twist the hair before curling.

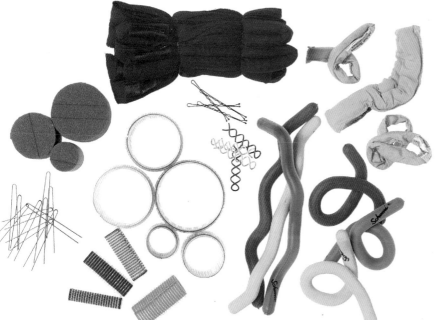

Left: Pin, clip, grip, roll, curl or tie – keep a supply of "extras" to hand for styling your hair.

Style Easy

The combination of practice and the right styling products enables you to achieve a salon finish at home. The products listed below will enable you to do it in style.

GELS

Gels come in varying degrees of viscosity, from a thick jelly to a liquid spray. They are sometimes called sculpting lotions and are used for precise styling. Use them to lift roots, tame wisps, create tendrils, calm static, heat set and give structure to curls. Wet gels can be used for sculpting styles.

HAIRSPRAY

Traditionally, hairspray was used to hold a style in place; today varying degrees of stiffness are available to suit all needs. Use hairspray to keep the hair in place, get curl definition when scrunching and mist over rollers when setting.

MOUSSE

Mousse is the most versatile styling product. It comes as a foam and can be used on wet or dry hair. Mousses contain conditioning agents and proteins to nurture and protect the hair. They are available in different strengths, designed to give soft to maximum holding power, and can be used to lift flat roots or smooth frizz. Use when blow-drying, scrunching and diffuser-drying.

SERUMS

Serums, glossers, polishes and shine sprays are made from oils or silicones, which improve shine and softness by forming a microscopic film on the surface of the hair. Formulations vary from light and silky to heavier ones with an oily feel. They smooth the cuticle, encouraging the tiny scales to lie flat and reflect the light, making the hair shine. Use to improve the feel of the hair, to combat static, de-frizz, add shine and gloss and to temporarily repair split ends.

STYLING OR SETTING LOTIONS

Styling lotions contain resins that form a film on the hair and aid setting and protect the hair from heat damage. There are formulations for dry, coloured or sensitized hair; others give volume and shine. Use for roller-setting, scrunching, blow-drying and natural drying.

Tip

If you are using a styling lotion for heat setting, look for formulations that offer thermal protection.

WAXES, POMADES AND CREAMS

These products are made from natural waxes, softened with other ingredients such as mineral oils and lanolin to make them pliable. Some pomades contain vegetable wax and oil to give gloss and sheen. Other formulations produce foam and are water soluble, and leave no residue. Use these products for controlling frizz and static.

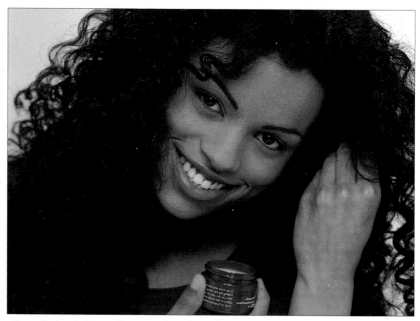

Above: Rub a little wax between the palms of your hands, then work into the curls with the fingertips to give separation and shine to thick, curly hair.

Appliances

Heated styling appliances allow you to style your hair quickly, efficiently and easily. A wide range of heated appliances is available.

AIR STYLERS

Air stylers combine the versatility of a hairdryer with the convenience of a styling wand. They operate on the same principle as a hairdryer, blowing warm air through the styler. Many come with a variety of clip-on options, including brushes, prongs and tongs. Use for creating waves and volume at the roots.

CRIMPERS

Crimpers consist of two ridged metal plates that produce uniform patterned crimps in straight lines in the hair. The hair must be straightened first, either by blow-drying or using flat irons. The crimper is then used to give waves or ripples. Use for special styling effects or to increase volume.

HAIRDRYERS

Choose a dryer that has a range of heat and speed settings so that the hair can be power-dried on high heat, finished on a lower heat, and then used with cool air to set the style. The life expectancy of a hairdryer averages between 200–300 hours. Use for blow-drying.

DIFFUSERS AND NOZZLES

Originally, diffusers were intended for drying curly hair, encouraging curl formation by spreading the airflow over the hair so the curls are not literally blown away. The prongs on the diffuser head also help to increase volume at the roots and give lift. Diffusers with flat heads are designed for gentle drying without ruffling and are more suitable for shorter styles. The newest type of diffuser has long, straight prongs that are designed to inject volume into straight hair while giving a smooth finish.

HEATED ROLLERS

A set of heated rollers will normally comprise a selection of 20 small, medium and large rollers, with colour-coded clips to match. Early models came with spikes, but newer developments include ribbed rubber surfaces, designed to be kinder to the hair.

The speed at which the rollers heat up varies, depending on the type of roller, but all rollers cool down completely in 30 minutes. Use heated rollers for quick sets, to give curl and body. They are ideal for preparing hair for dressing into styles.

Tip

Heat drying encourages static, causing hair to fly away. Reduce static by lightly touching your hair, or mist your hair brush with hairspray to calm the hair.

Below: Rollers make great styling tools.

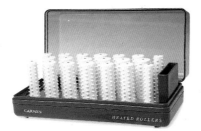

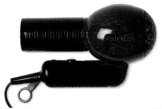

Above: Hairdryers are an essential piece of equipment for quick-drying and styling hair.

STRAIGHTENERS

Straighteners are similar to crimpers but have flat plates to iron out frizz or curl. Use for "pressing" really curly hair.

TONGS

Tongs consist of a barrel, or prong, and a depressor groove. The thickness of the barrel varies, and the size of the tong that is used depends on whether small, medium or large curls are required.

HOT BRUSHES

Hot brushes are easier to handle than tongs and come in varying sizes for creating curls of different sizes. Wind down the lengths of the hair, hold for a few seconds until the heat has penetrated through the hair, then gently remove. Cordless hot brushes use gas cartridges or batteries to produce heat and are used to give root lift, curl and movement.

TRAVEL DRYERS

Travel dryers are ideal for taking on holiday. They are usually miniature versions of standard dryers, and some are even available with their own small diffusers. Check that the dryer you buy has dual voltage and a travel case.

Blow-drying

Follow our step-by-step sequence for the smoothest, sleekest blow-dried hairstyle ever.

Styling Checklist
You will need:
styling comb
hairdryer
mousse
clip
styling brush
serum

1 Shampoo and condition your hair, as usual. Comb through gently with a wide-toothed comb to remove any tangles.

2 Partially dry your hair to remove excess moisture. Apply a handful of mousse to the palm of your hand. Using your other hand, spread the mousse through the hair, distributing it evenly from the tips to the ends.

3 Divide your hair into two sections by clipping the top and sides out of the way. Then, working on the hair that is left free and taking one small section at a time, hold the dryer in one hand and a styling brush in the other. Place the brush underneath the first section of hair, positioning it at the roots. Keeping the tension on the hair taut, move the brush towards the end, directing the air flow from the dryer so that it follows the downwards movement of the brush.

4 Curve the brush under at the ends to achieve a slight bend. Concentrate on drying the root area first, repeatedly introducing the brush to the roots once it has moved down the length of the hair. Continue the movement until the first section of the hair is dry. Repeat step 4 until the whole of the back section is dry.

5 Release a section of hair from the top and dry it in the same manner. Continue in this way until you have dried all your hair. Finish by smoothing a few drops of serum through the hair to flatten any flyaway ends.

Tips
■ Use the highest heat setting to remove excess moisture, then switch to medium to finish drying.
■ Point the air flow downwards. This smoothes the cuticles and makes the hair shine.
■ Make sure each section is dry before going on to the next.

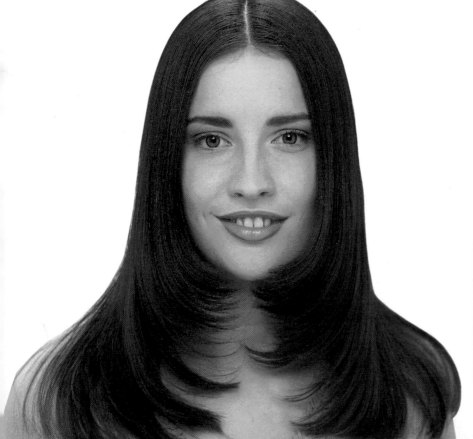

Roll-Up

Roller sets form the basis of many hairstyles; use them to smooth hair, add waves or soft curls, or to provide a foundation for an upswept style.

1 Shampoo and condition your hair, then partially dry to remove excess moisture. Mist with a styling lotion.

2 For a basic set, take a 5 cm/2 in section of hair (or a section the same width as your roller) from the centre front and comb it straight up, smoothing out any tangles. Wrap the ends of the sectioned hair around the roller, taking care not to buckle the hair. Then wind the roller down firmly, towards the scalp, keeping the tension even and comfortably taut.

3 Keep winding until the roller sits at the roots of the hair. Self-fixing rollers will stay in place on their own, but if you are using brush rollers you will have to fasten them with a pin.

4 Continue around the whole head, always taking the same width of hair. Re-mist the hair with styling lotion if it begins to dry out.

5 Leave the finished set to dry naturally, or dry it with a diffuser attachment on your hand dryer, or with a hood dryer. If using artificial heat sources let the dry hair cool before you remove the rollers. Brush through the hair following the direction of the set. Mist the brush with hairspray and use to smooth any stray hairs.

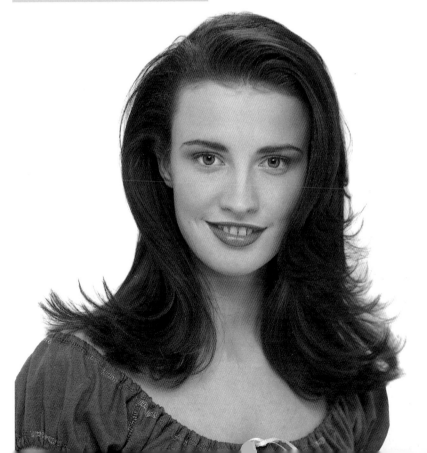

Tips
■ Use large diameter rollers for sleek, wavy looks, smaller rollers for curlier styles.
■ Always use sections of equal width when setting your hair or you will get an uneven result.
■ For maximum volume and control, let the hair cool down completely before brushing through.
■ A bristle brush will give a smoother finish to the style.
■ If the finished set is too curly after brushing through, loosen the curl with a brush used with a hand dryer.
■ To create extra volume and height use a fine-toothed comb to backcomb the roots.

Finger-drying

This is a quick method of drying and styling your hair. It relies on the heat released from your hands rather than the heat from a dryer. Finger-drying is suitable for short to mid-length hair.

Styling Checklist
You will need:
spray gel
styling comb

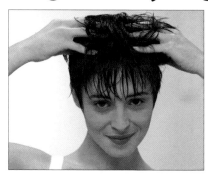

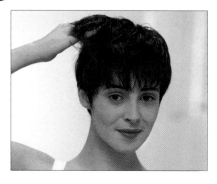

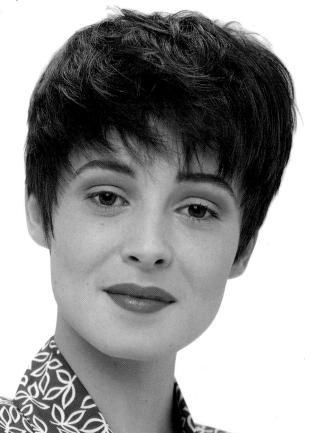

1 Shampoo and condition your hair as usual, then spray with gel and comb through gently.

2 Run your fingers upwards and forwards, from the roots to the ends.

3 Lift the hair at the crown to get height at the roots.

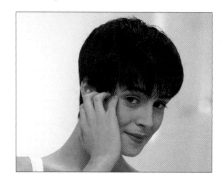

4 Continue lifting as the hair dries. Use your fingertips to flatten the hair at the sides.

Tip
Finger-drying is the best way to dry damaged hair or to encourage waves in naturally curly, short hair.

Barrel Curls

One of the simplest sets is achieved by curling the hair around the fingers and then pinning the curl in place. Barrel curls create a soft set.

1 Shampoo and condition your hair; apply setting lotion and comb through from the roots to the ends. Take a small section of hair (about 2.5 cm/1 in) and smooth it upwards.

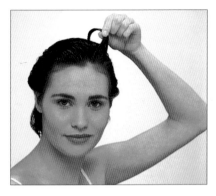

2 Loop the hair into a large curl.

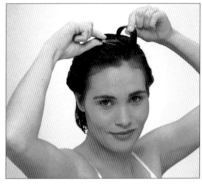

3 Clip the curl in place.

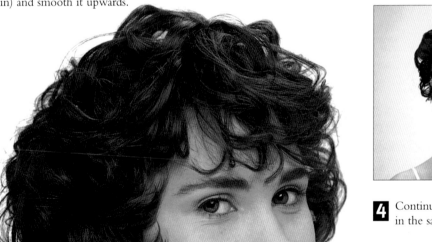

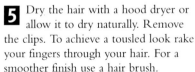

4 Continue to curl the rest of the hair in the same way.

5 Dry the hair with a hood dryer or allow it to dry naturally. Remove the clips. To achieve a tousled look rake your fingers through your hair. For a smoother finish use a hair brush.

Soft-setting

Fabric rollers are the modern version of old-fashioned rags. Apart from being very easy to use they are kind to the hair and give a highly effective set.

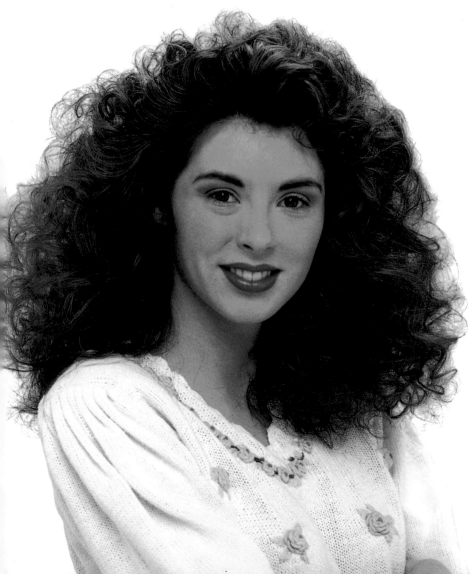

Styling Checklist
You will need:
styling lotion
fabric rollers

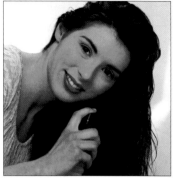

1 Dampen the hair with styling lotion, making sure you distribute it evenly from the roots to the ends.

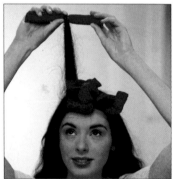

2 Using sections of hair about 2.5 cm/1 in wide, curl the end of the hair around a fabric roller and wind the roller down towards the scalp, taking care not to buckle the ends of the hair.

Tip
For even more volume, twist each section of hair lengthwise before winding it on to the fabric roller.

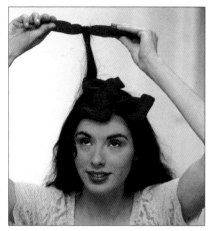

3 Continue winding the roller right down to the roots.

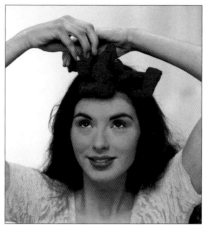

4 To fasten, simply bend each end of the fabric roller towards the centre. This grips the hair and holds it in place.

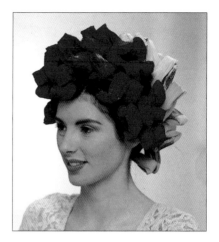

5 Leave to dry naturally when the complete set of rollers is in place.

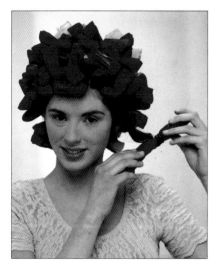

6 When the hair is dry, remove the rollers by unbending the ends and unwinding the hair.

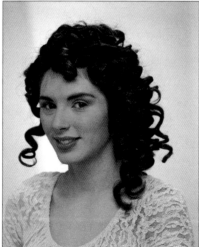

7 When all the rollers have been removed the hair falls into firm corkscrew curls.

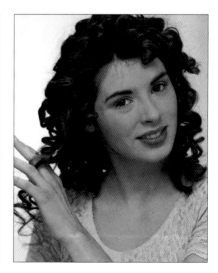

8 Working on one curl at a time, rake your fingers through the hair, teasing out each curl. The result will be a full, voluminous finish.

Tong and Twist

Tongs can be used to smooth the hair and add just the right amount of movement.

1 Shampoo, condition and dry your hair. Apply a mist of styling lotion. Never use mousse as it will stick to the tongs and bake into the hair. Divide off a small section of hair.

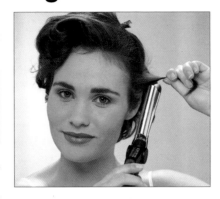

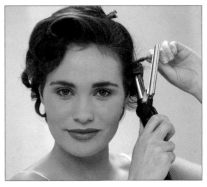

2 Press the depressor to open the tongs.

3 Wind the section of hair around the barrel of the tongs.

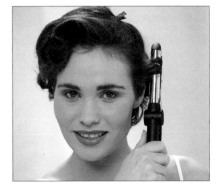

4 Release the depressor to hold the hair in place and wait a few seconds for the curl to form. Remove the tongs and leave the hair to cool while you work on the rest of your hair. Style by raking through with your fingers.

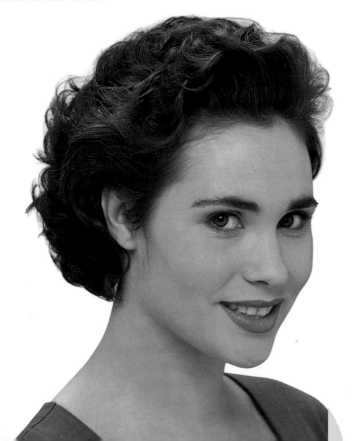

Airwaves

Air styling makes use of gentle heat and combines it with the moisture in your hair to give a long lasting curl.

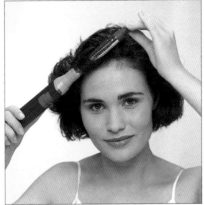

---

1 Shampoo and condition your hair. Mist with styling lotion.

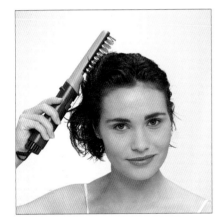

2 Using the brush attachment on the styler, start drying the hair. Lift each section to allow the heat to dry the roots.

Tip
Switch your air styler to low speed for more controlled styling and finishing.

---

3 Clip on the tong attachment and continue shaping the hair by wrapping it around the tongs.

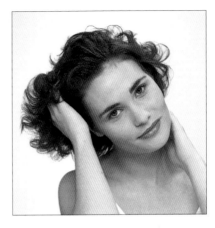

4 Repeat steps 2 and 3 until the whole head is curled and waved. When the hair is completely dry rake your fingers through it.

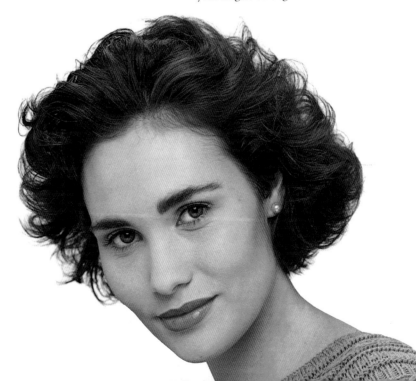

Dragged Side Braids

Curly hair can be controlled, yet still allowed to flow free, by braiding it at the sides and allowing the hair at the back to fall in a mass of curls.

Styling Checklist
Time: 5 minutes
Ease/Difficulty: Easy
Hair type: Long and naturally curly or permed
You will need:
styling comb
covered bands
hair grips

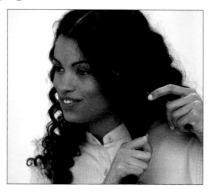

1 Part your hair in the centre and divide off a large section at the side, combing it as flat as possible to the head.

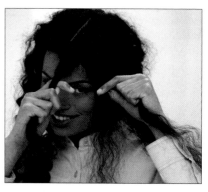

2 Divide the section into three equal strands and hold them apart.

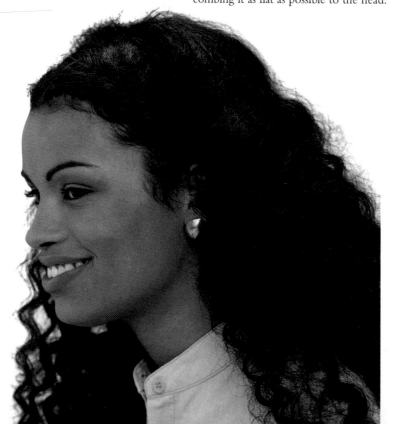

3 Make a dragged braid by pulling the strands of hair towards your face and then taking the right strand over the centre strand, the left strand over the centre, and the right over the centre again, keeping the braid in position.

4 Continue braiding to the end and secure the end with a covered band. Tuck the braid behind your ear and grip it in place, then make a second braid on the other side.

Ribbon Bow

Asimple ponytail is given added interest by binding with ribbon and finishing with a bow.

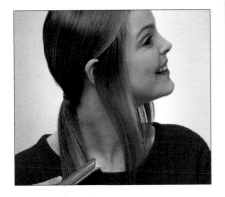

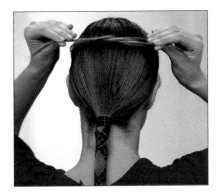

3 Cross the ribbon over the ponytail, continuing until you are 5–7.5 cm/ 2–3 in from the end. Tie the ribbon into a bow. Smooth out the side sections of hair and tie them into a neat bow at the centre back of your head above the be-ribboned ponytail. Secure with a hairpin if necessary.

1 Brush or comb your hair smoothly back into a neat ponytail, leaving a small section free at either side. Secure the ponytail with a covered band.

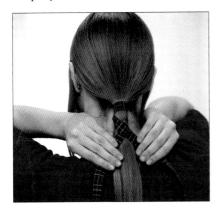

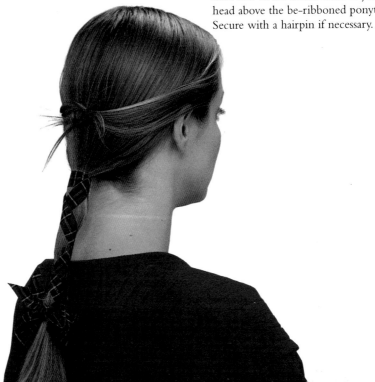

2 Position the centre of the ribbon over the band as shown, pulling the ends of the ribbon taut.

Ponytail Styler

A simple ponytail can be transformed into something very sophisticated using this clever styler.

Styling Checklist

Time: 10–15 minutes, depending on experience
Ease/difficulty: Quite easy, but can be fiddly
Hair type: Long, straight, one length
You will need:
covered band
ponytail styler

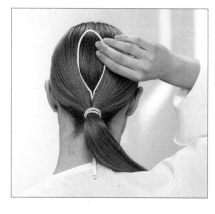

1 Clasp the hair into a neat ponytail and secure it with a covered band. Insert the styler as shown.

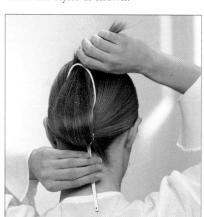

2 Pull the ponytail up and thread it through the styler.

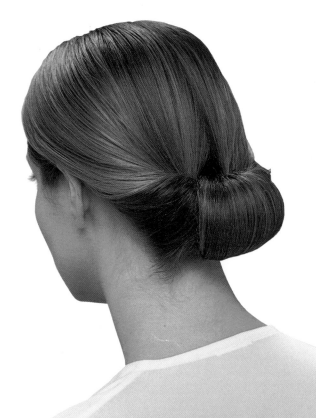

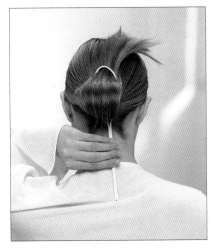

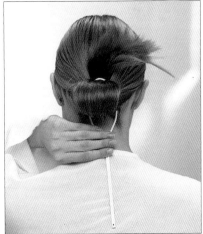

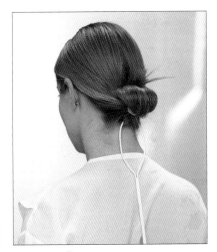

3 Begin to pull the styler down . . .

4 . . . continue pulling . . .

5 . . . so the ponytail pulls through . . .

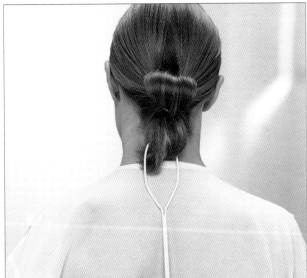

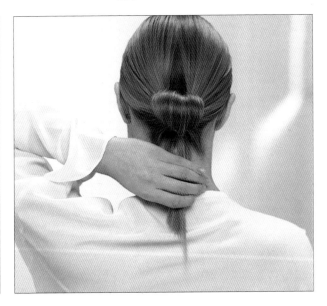

6 . . . and emerges underneath.

7 Smooth the hair with your hand and insert the styler again, repeating steps 2 to 6 once more to give a neat and smooth chignon loop.

Curly Styler

The ponytail styler can also be used to tame a mass of curls, creating a ponytail with a simple double twist.

Tip
When inserting the styler through a ponytail, carefully move it from side to side in order to create enough room to pull the looped end of the styler through more easily.

Styling Checklist
Time: 5 minutes
Ease/difficulty: Easy
Hair type: Long and naturally curly or permed.
You will need:
widely spaced tooth comb
covered band
ponytail styler
mousse

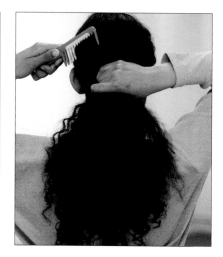

1 Use a comb with widely spaced teeth to smooth the hair back and into a ponytail. Secure with a covered hair band.

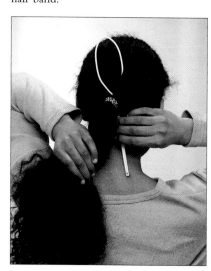

2 Insert the styler as shown.

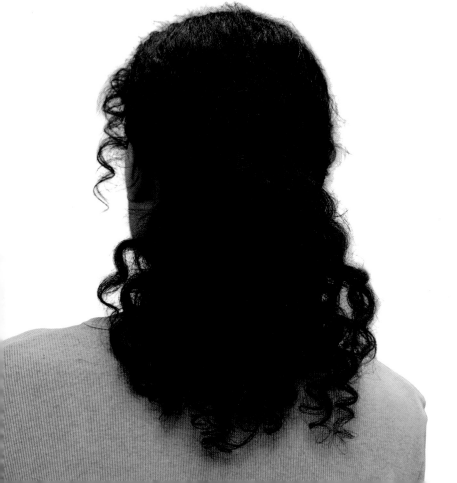

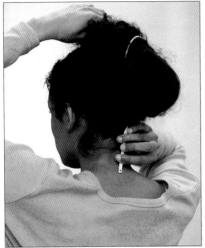

3 Pull the ponytail up and thread it through the styler.

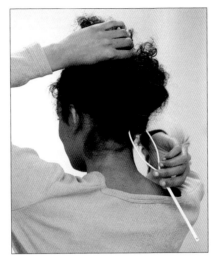

4 Begin to pull the styler down . . .

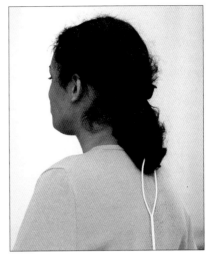

5 . . . continue pulling . . .

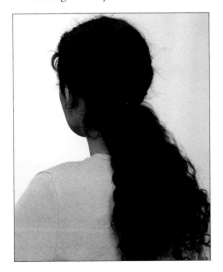

6 . . . so that the ponytail pulls all the way through.

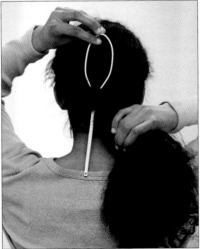

7 Repeat steps 2 to 6.

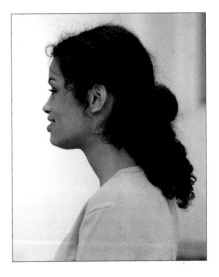

8 Apply a little mousse to your hands and use it to re-form the curls, scrunching to achieve a good shape.

French Braid

This elegant, sophisticated braid looks complicated but it does get easier with practice.

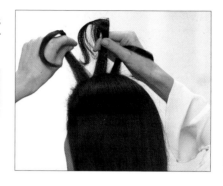

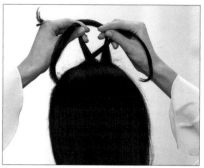

Styling Checklist

Time: 15–20 minutes
Ease/difficulty: Quite difficult
Hair type: Mid-length to long and straight
You will need:
covered band
scrunchie

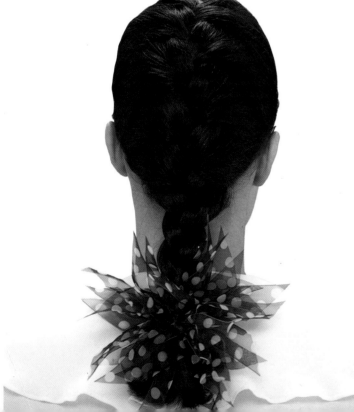

1 Take a section of hair from the front of the head and divide into three even strands. Braid once, taking the left and right strands over the centre strand.

2 Hold the braid and use your thumbs to gather additional hair (approximately 1 cm/½ in strips) from each side of the head. Add these to the original strands. Braid the strands once again.

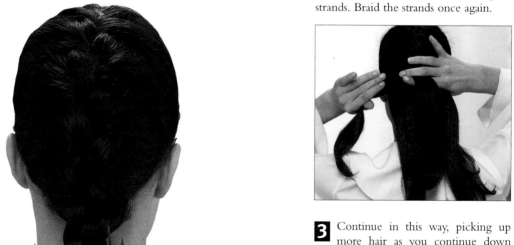

3 Continue in this way, picking up more hair as you continue down the braid. Secure the French braid with a covered band and add a scrunchie.

Tip
Shorter front layers can be woven into this type of braid, as when growing out a fringe, for example.

Double-stranded Braids

These clever braids have a fishbone pattern, which gives an unusual look.

Styling Checklist
Time: 10 minutes
Ease/difficulty: Needs practice
Hair type: Long and straight
You will need:
styling comb
covered bands
coloured feathers
two short lengths of fine leather

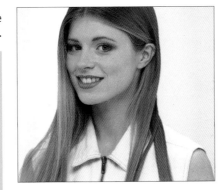

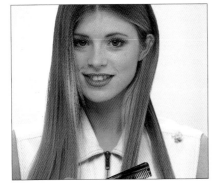

1 Part your hair in the centre and comb it straight.

2 Divide the hair on one side of your head into two strands, then take a fine section from the back of the back strand and take it over to join the front strand, as shown.

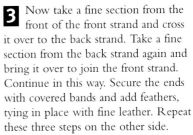

3 Now take a fine section from the front of the front strand and cross it over to the back strand. Take a fine section from the back strand again and bring it over to join the front strand. Continue in this way. Secure the ends with covered bands and add feathers, tying in place with fine leather. Repeat these three steps on the other side.

Crown Braids

By braiding the crown hair and allowing the remaining hair to frame the face you can achieve an interesting contrast of textures.

Styling Checklist
Time: 15 minutes
Ease/difficulty: Needs practice
Hair type: Mid-length to long and naturally curly or permed
You will need:
large clip
styling comb
small covered bands
Alice headband

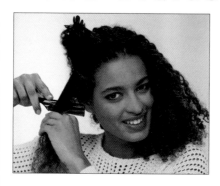

1 Clip up the top hair on one side of your head, leaving the back hair free. Take a small section of hair at ear level and comb it straight.

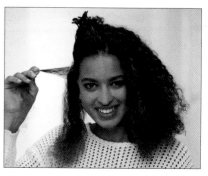

2 Start braiding quite tightly, doing one cross (right strand over centre, left over centre), and gradually bring more hair into the outside strands.

3 Continue in this way, taking the braid towards the back of the head.

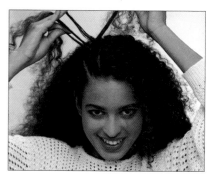

4 Make another parting about 2.5 cm/1 in parallel to and above the previous braid, and repeat the process. Continue in this way until all the front hair has been braided. Secure the braids with small covered bands and scrunch the remaining hair into large curls to increase the volume. Finally, add a decorative Alice band.

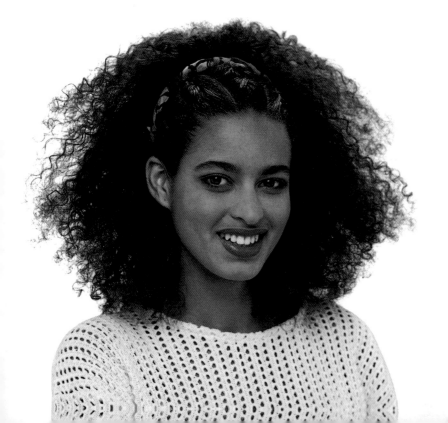

Rick-rack Braids

You can achieve a colourful look by braiding the hair with rick-rack to give a young, fresh style.

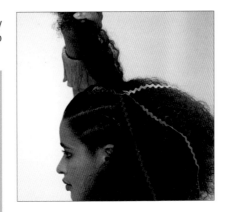

2 Take a section of hair and divide it into three strands, aligning one piece of rick-rack with each strand.

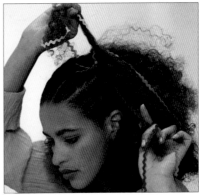

3 Begin braiding, taking the right strand over the centre strand, the left over the centre, right over the centre, and so on. Continue braiding down to the ends, add small covered bands and tie the rick-rack to fasten.

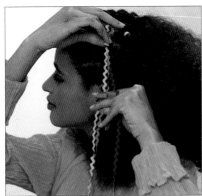

1 Braid the front of the hair. Tie three strands of rick-rack at one end and pin to the band of one braid.

Tip
Naturally curly or permed hair benefits from regular intensive conditioning treatments.

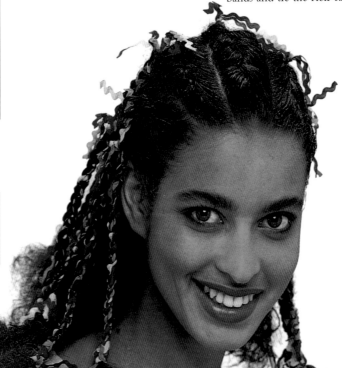

Basketweave Braid

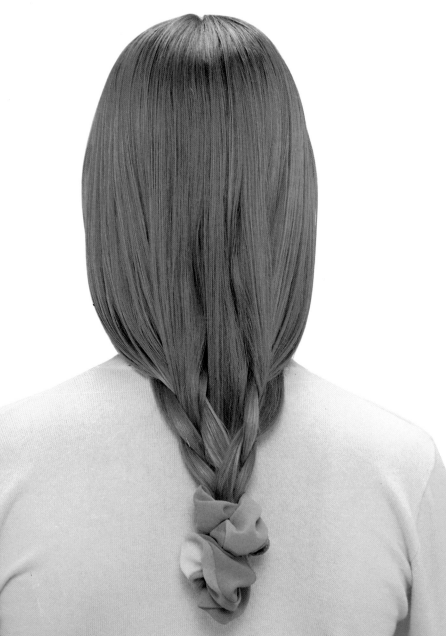

Enlist the help of a friend to help you create this unusual braid style.

Styling Checklist

Time: 10 minutes
Ease/difficulty: Needs practice
Hair type: Mid-length to long
You will need:
styling comb
scrunchie

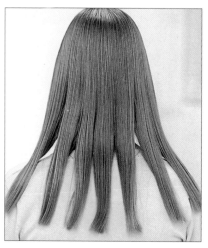

1 Divide the hair into seven equal strands – three strands on either side of the face and one at the centre back.

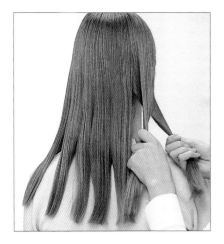

2 Starting at the right-hand side, cross the first strand (the strand nearest the face) over the second strand.

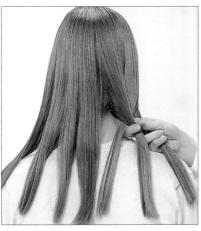

3 Cross the third strand over what is now the second strand, as shown.

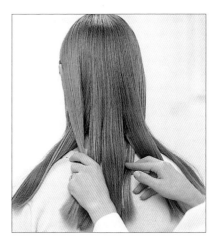

4 Repeat steps 2 and 3 on the left side. What was originally the first strand in each group will now be the third strand.

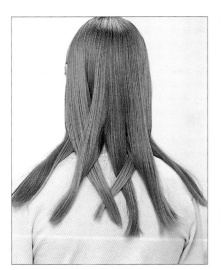

5 Take the third strand on the right-hand side over the central strand, and under the third strand on the left-hand side.

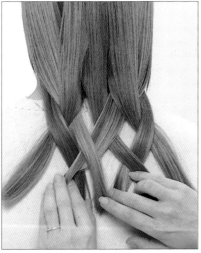

6 Now bring the first strand on the right-hand side over the second strand and under the central strand.

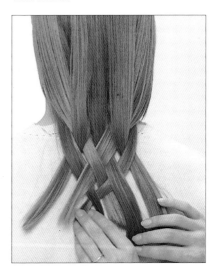

7 Repeat step 6 on the left side. Finally, clasp with a scrunchie to secure in place.

Twist and Coil

This style starts with a simple ponytail, is easy to do and looks stunning.

Styling Checklist
Time: 10 minutes
Ease/difficulty: Easy
Hair type: Long, one length, straight hair
You will need:
small covered band
shine spray
hairpins
1 m/1 yd strip of sequins

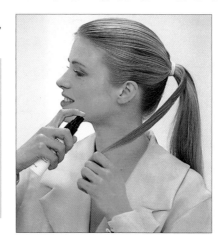

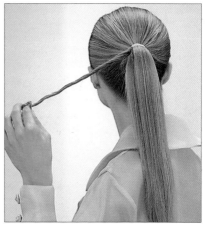

1 Brush the hair and smooth it back, securing it in a ponytail using a small covered band.

2 Divide off a section of hair and mist with shine spray for some gloss.

3 Holding the ends of a section, twist the hair until it rolls back on itself to form a coil.

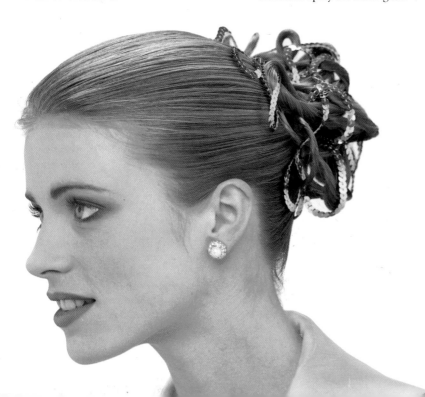

4 Position the coil in a loop as shown and secure in place using hairpins. Continue in this manner until all the hair has been coiled. Decorate by intertwining with a strip of sequins.

Cameo Braid

Aclassic bun is given extra panache by encircling it with a braid.

1 Smooth the hair into a ponytail, leaving one section of the hair free.

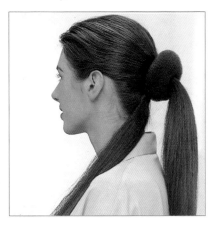

2 Place a bun ring over the ponytail.

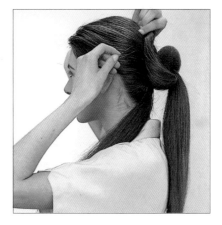

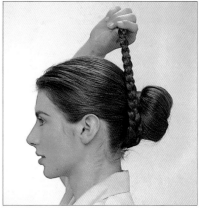

3 Take approximately one-third of the hair from the ponytail and wrap it around the bun ring, securing with pins. Repeat with the other two-thirds of the hair.

4 Braid the section of hair that was left out of the ponytail, right strand over centre strand, left over centre and so on, and wrap the braid around the base of the bun, then secure with pins.

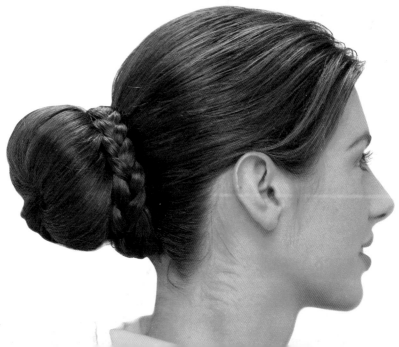

Rope Braid

A simple braid is entwined with rope to give an unusual finish.

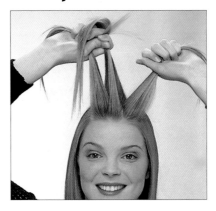

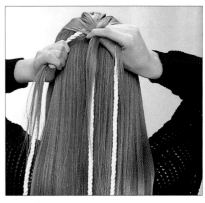

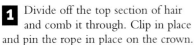 Divide off the top section of hair and comb it through. Clip in place and pin the rope in place on the crown.

2 Separate the front piece of hair into three equal strands. Begin to braid.

3 When the braid reaches the top of the rope, merge a strand of rope with each strand of braid and continue working down to the ends.

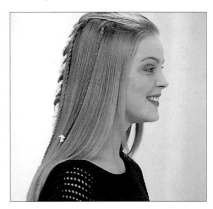

4 Secure with a covered band. Then make four more small braids, equally spaced around the head, and secure each end with covered bands.

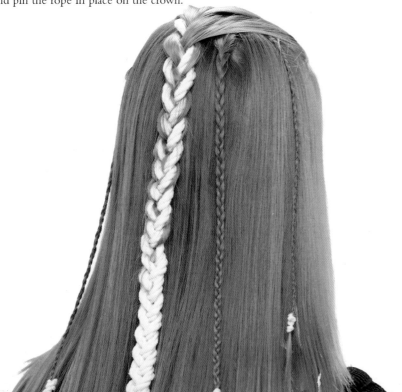

City Slicker

Transform your hair in a matter of minutes into this punchy young style, using gel to slick it into shape.

Styling Checklist
Time: 5 minutes
Ease/difficulty: Easy
Hair type: Short crops
You will need:
sculpting gel
small vent brush
styling comb

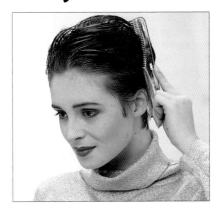

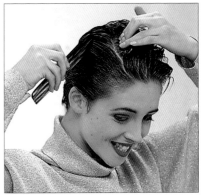

1 Take a generous amount of gel and apply it to the hair from the roots down to the ends.

3 Comb the hair into shape using a styling comb to give movement.

4 Shape the hair to form a quiff and sleek down the sides and back.

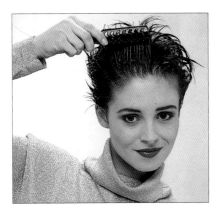

2 Use a vent brush, a comb or your fingers to distribute the gel evenly through the hair.

Tip
Make sure you distribute the gel evenly all over your hair before styling.

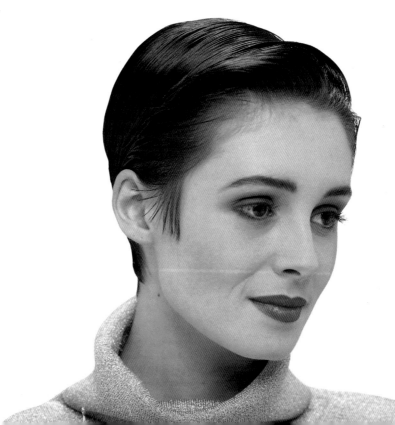

Mini Braids

This fresh and upbeat look is an ideal style for teenagers.

Styling Checklist
Time: Rather time consuming
Ease/difficulty: Needs practice
Hair type: Long and straight
You will need:
styling wax
small covered bands
a length of ribbon about 1 m/1 yd
long, cut into 6 pieces

Tip
To smooth any flyaway ends
rub a few drops of serum between
the palms of your hands and
smooth over the hair.

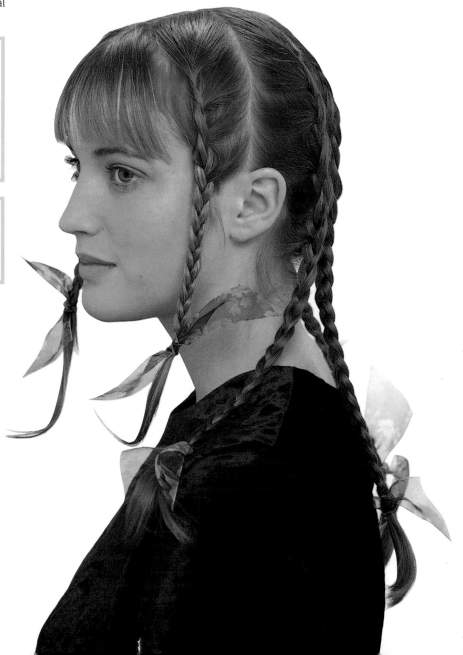

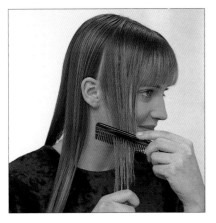

1 Part the hair in the centre and smooth with a little wax that has first been warmed between the palms of your hands before spreading over the hair.

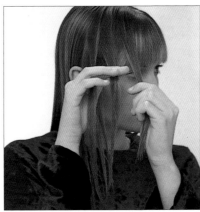

2 Divide off a section at one side, as shown, and divide again into three equal parts.

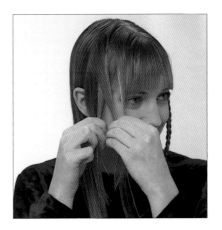

3 Braid the hair by placing the right strand over the centre strand, the left over the centre, right over the centre, and so on, pulling the braid slightly towards the face.

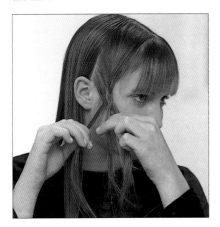

4 Continue down to the ends of the hair and secure with a small covered band. Repeat on the other side.

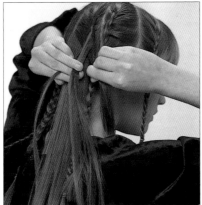

5 Part the back hair into four equal sections, from the crown down to the nape, and braid as shown. Start the braid at the top with three strands of hair and, after each turn of the braid, add a small section from each side.

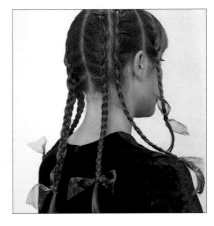

6 Secure the ends of the braids with small covered bands and decorate the braids with ribbon bows.

Band Braid

Aplain ponytail can be transformed beyond recognition by simply covering the band with a tiny braid.

Styling Checklist
Time: 5 minutes
Ease/difficulty: Easy
Hair type: Long, one length
You will need:
styling brush
styling wax
small covered band
hair grips

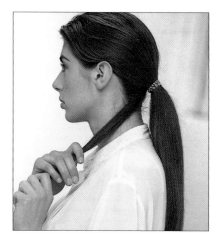

1 Brush the hair into a ponytail and secure with a band, leaving a small section free for braiding. Smooth the section with styling wax.

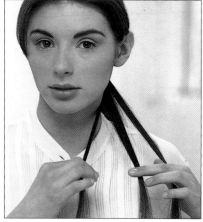

2 Divide this section into three equal strands. Now, braid the hair in the normal way.

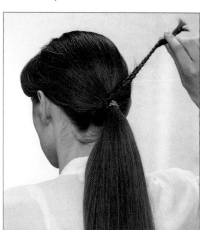
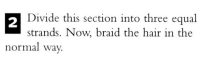

3 Take the braid and wrap it around the covered band as many times as it goes. Secure the braid in place with hair grips.

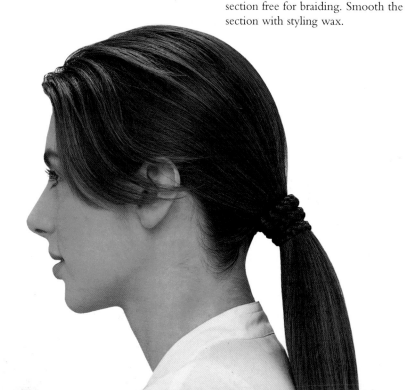

Draped Chignon

This elegant style is perfect for that special evening out.

Styling Checklist
Time: 5–10 minutes
Ease/difficulty: Quite easy
Hair type: Long and straight
You will need:
styling comb
small covered bands
hair grips

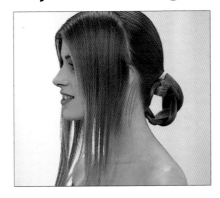

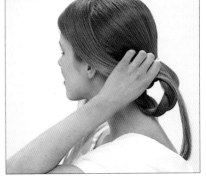

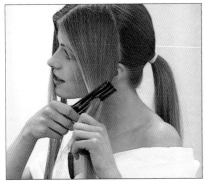

2 Loosely braid the ponytail – take the right strand over the centre strand, the left over the right, the right over the centre, and so on, continuing to the end. Secure the end with a small band, then tuck the end under and around in a loop and secure with grips.

3 Pick up the hair on the left side and comb it in a curve back to the ponytail loop. Swirl this hair over and under the loop and secure with grips. Repeat step 3 on the right side.

1 Part the hair in the centre from the forehead to the middle of the crown. Comb the side hair and scoop the back hair into a low ponytail using a covered band.

Tip
Long hair should be trimmed at least every two months to keep it in good condition.

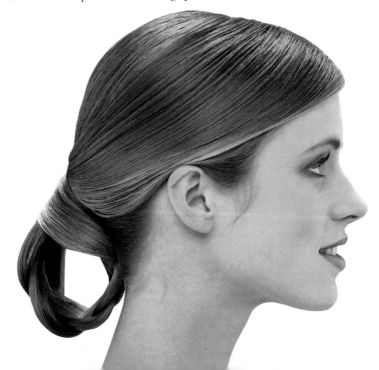

Simple Pleat

Curly hair that is neatly pleated makes a sophisticated style. The front is left full to soften the effect.

Styling Checklist
Time: 5 minutes
Ease/difficulty: Quite easy
Hair type: Shoulder length or longer
You will need:
serum
hairpins

1 Divide off a section of hair at the front and leave it free. Smooth with serum. Take the remaining hair into one hand, as if making a ponytail. Twist the hair tightly, the length of the ponytail, from left to right.

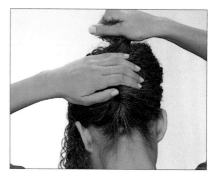

2 When the twist is taut, turn the hair upwards as shown to form a pleat. Use your other hand to help smooth the pleat and at the same time neaten the top by tucking in the ends.

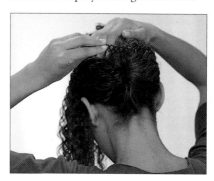

3 Secure the pleat with hairpins. Take the reserved front section, bring it back and secure at the top of the pleat, allowing the ends to fall free.

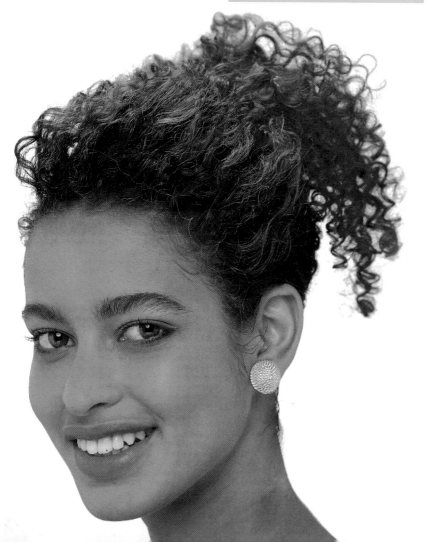

Looped Curls

Two ponytails form the basis of this elegant style.

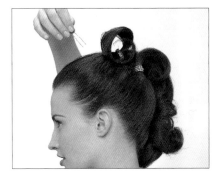

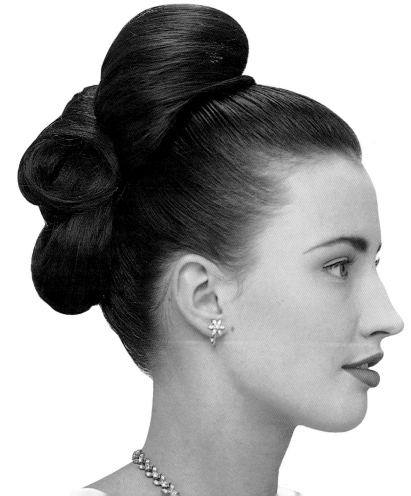

3 Divide each ponytail into sections about 2.5 cm/1 in wide, then comb and smooth each section into a looped curl and pin in place. Set with hairspray.

Tip
The speed at which rollers heat up depend on the type of roller, so check the instructions of your own model.

1 Apply setting lotion to the ends of the hair to help form bouncy curls. Set the hair on heated rollers for the required amount of time. When the rollers are cool – about 10 minutes after completing the set – take them out and allow the hair to fall free.

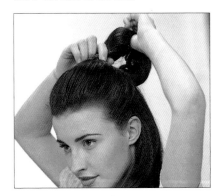

2 Divide off the crown hair and secure it with hair pins in a high ponytail. Apply a few drops of serum to add gloss, and brush the hair through. Place the remaining hair in a lower ponytail.

French Pleat

Mid-length to long hair can be trans-formed into a classic, elegant French pleat in a matter of minutes.

Styling Checklist

Time: 5–10 minutes
Ease/difficulty: Quite easy
Hair type: Mid-length to long
You will need:
styling comb
hair grips
hairpins
hairspray

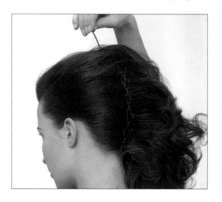

1 Backcomb the hair all over, then smooth it across to the centre back. Form the centre by criss-crossing hair grips from the crown downwards.

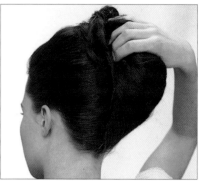

2 Gently smooth the hair around from the other side, leaving the front section free, and tuck the ends under to neaten.

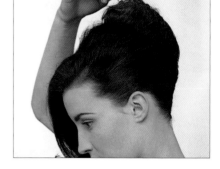

3 Secure with pins, then lightly comb the front section up and around to merge with the top of the pleat. Mist with hairspray to hold the style in place.

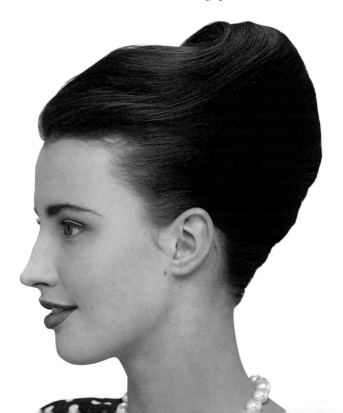

Short and Spiky

Short hair can be quickly styled using gel and wax to create a bold and fun look for instant glamour.

Styling Checklist
Time: 10 minutes
Ease/difficulty: Easy
Hair type: Short, layered and straight
You will need:
styling gel
hairdryer
styling comb
styling wax

1 Work styling gel through your hair from the roots to the ends.

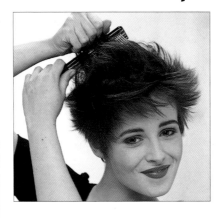

3 When the hair is dry, backcomb the crown to give additional height.

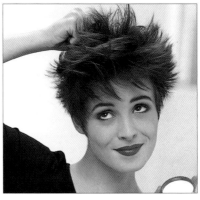

4 To finish, rub a little wax between the palms of your hands, then apply it to the hair to give definition.

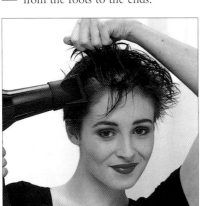
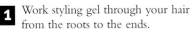

2 Dry your hair using a directional nozzle on your dryer; as you dry, lift sections of the hair to create height.

Tip
Gel can be reactivated by misting the hair with water and shaping it into style again.

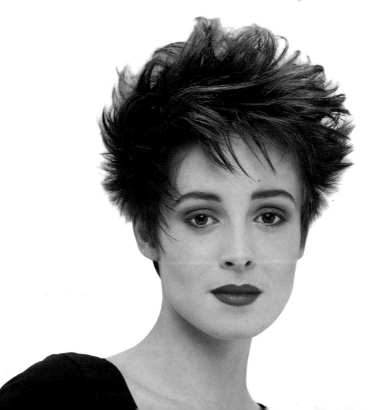

Accessories

Nothing becomes a hairstyle quite like hair accessories. Bandeaux, ribbons and bows come into their own at party time, but they can also be used at any time to transform your hair – instantly.

MAKE YOUR OWN

Some pretty fabrics and materials for hair accessories can be found in haberdashery departments of large stores. Look out for strips of sequins and pearls, or choose pretty ribbons, multi-coloured beads and tiny embroidered flowers that can be tied or simply pinned into place.

SCRUNCHIES

Scrunchies are elasticated bands that are covered with a tube of fabric, which ruches up when it is placed over a ponytail. They are available in a wide variety of fabrics, including fine pleated silks, velvets and soft chiffons, so you can wear them to match your outfit.

BEADS

Beads can be threaded on to strands of hair and secured with small bands for special looks. You could revamp old clips and slides by adding your own beads to make some fun and original accessories.

BENDIES

Bendies are long pieces of flexible wire encased in fabric – often velvet or silk – that can be twisted into the hair in a variety of eye-catching ways; for example as a band, braided into a ponytail, entwined round a bun, or bound on to a braid. They come in many different colours and materials.

FLOWERS

For special occasions such as weddings, fresh flowers attached to clips make the perfect decoration. If you want to keep your floral accessories for longer, use silk flowers instead.

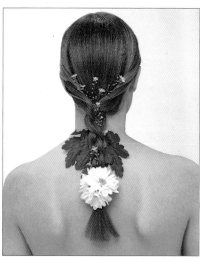

Above: Fresh flowers can be pinned into any braided style.

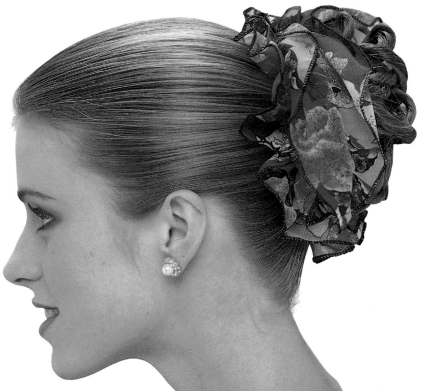

Left: A scrunchie completely alters the appearance of the Twist and Coil style.

BOWS

Bows can be tailored or floppy and are usually made from soft silks and velvets attached to a slide. Bows are available in a wide range of colours and designs.

HEADBANDS

Headbands come in a wide variety of fabrics and widths. Classic colours such as black, navy, red, cream and tortoise-shell are good basics.

SLIDES, CHIGNON PINS, COMBS

Unusual slides and barrettes are excellent for finishing off a braid or adding interest to a ponytail. Chignon pins add instant sophistication and are a means of securing buns. Combs can be used to lift the hair off the face, allowing the hair to fall free, but not in your eyes.

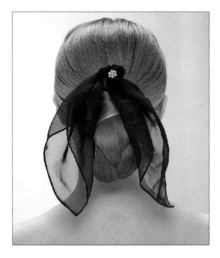

Above: A floppy bow adds instant sparkle to the Ponytail Styler.

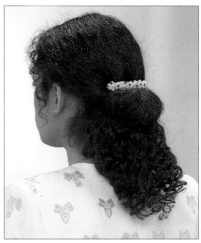

Above: A pearl slide gives added interest to the Curly Styler.

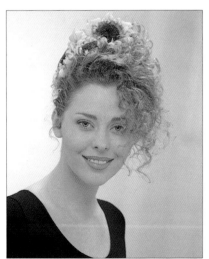

Above: Pin artificial flowers on top of an upswept style or into loosely styled curly hair for a young and very natural look.

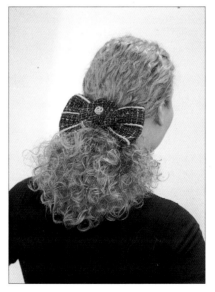

Above: For a very feminine touch add a pretty bow slide.

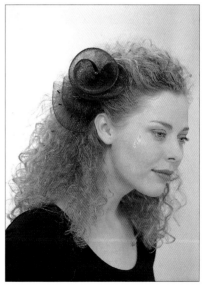

Above: For the evening, clip a classic bow among the curls.

Index

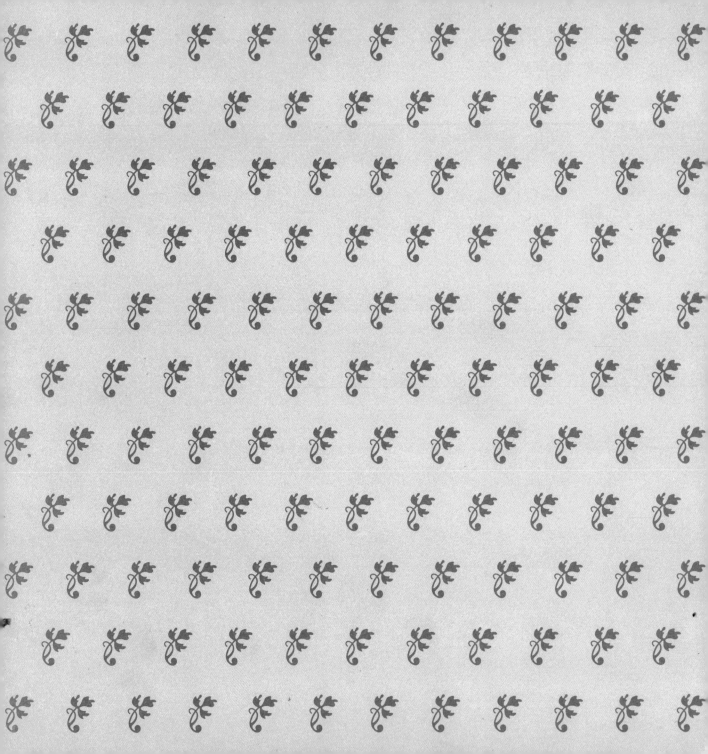